LARGER THAN LIFE

Larger Than
LIFE

From Childhood Abuse to
Celebrity Weight-Loss TV Show

Bruce Pitcher

with Rachel Sommer

Designed and Typeset by Timm Bryson, em em design, LLC

Library of Congress Control Number: 2018952431

ISBN 978-1-7320954-0-3 (paperback)
ISBN 978-1-7320954-1-0 (e-book)

10 9 8 7 6 5 4 3 2 1

To all the victims, you are not alone.

CONTENTS

FOREWORD

When we met Bruce for the first time, he was full of personality. He told hilarious jokes, was the first to talk in every situation, and rallied everyone around him during the workouts. We had seen this personality before, and to be honest, we were unsure that he was truly ready to transform.

It is very common for someone who is feeling inadequate in some aspects of their life to overcompensate in others: achievements, possessions, power, and in Bruce's case, a boisterous personality.

This 'masking' is basic human behavior 101. So right off the bat, we were a bit skeptical.

So it turned into a waiting game for us. People can only keep a mask on for so long. After a few weeks, especially as we dig into the emotional side of transformation, we typically get a glimpse of everyone's true character. But day after day, week after week, Bruce remained steadfast.

He remained passionate and driven. He laughed, he cried, he shared openly and never held back. He became a reluctant leader among the others, as everyone naturally gravitated toward him to draw inspiration and motivation when they struggled to find it within themselves.

Bruce was different. He was special.

What makes Bruce truly extraordinary is not just his passion or ability to motivate others. What makes him so special
is that he harnesses a courage within that we have never seen
before in any human. He is so brave as to allow himself to be
vulnerable—even in threatening times.

This rare quality makes him a man among men. His selfless courage to be vulnerable and open gives permission to
everyone around him to do the same. This is a place where
so many refuse to go, in fear of looking bad or looking weak
in front of others. But Bruce has found that this is the magic
that truly heals the soul and changes lives—starting with his
own.

Over our year with Bruce, we witnessed firsthand the
most beautiful expression of love and forgiveness... even
in the most unthinkable circumstances. Not only did he
deeply impact our lives and our outlook on the world, but
he made a lasting impact on everyone who was blessed to
spend a year with him—the producers, cameramen, support
staff—everyone.

His shining example of love, forgiveness, and self-
actualization have been a beacon of hope for thousands. And
he can certainly add us to the list of people whose lives he
has changed forever.

We are beyond excited for you to meet Bruce and read his
story. You'll see that we all need a little Bruce in our lives!

—*Chris and Heidi Powell*

PREFACE

When I heard Bruce's story, I wanted to help him share it because I knew whoever read it would be changed. Little did I know that I would be changed most of all.

I began talking with Bruce on the phone every day for several weeks, hearing his story. What he has overcome brought me to tears, and not just once. Often, after hanging up from our daily talks, or working on a particularly gruesome chapter, or reading over the court documents, I would cry. My heart broke thinking about something so horrific happening to anyone.

However, as often as I felt overcome by the evil that was inflicted on an innocent boy, I was also inspired by Bruce. No normal human being should have the positive outlook he has on life after going through what he went through. It was Bruce who would keep me going every day. It was Bruce who showed me what hard work and dedication can be. It was Bruce who opened my eyes and my heart to what forgiveness really looks like. This guy is INCREDIBLE.

The man is so humble that I didn't really understand the magnitude of the impact he leaves everywhere he goes until I started the interviews. It was an absolute delight talking to his friends and family because they all spoke so enthusiastically about this unrelenting, positive person. Bruce doesn't give up on anyone or anything. His example pushes me every day to develop that within myself.

I don't know how to thank Bruce for the gift he has given me. But I know he is a miracle, a miracle the world should know about.

—*Rachel Sommer*

Introduction

'm so sick of hearing those statistics!

That's how I felt before I lost over 200 pounds on ABC's *Extreme Weight Loss*. I used to weigh 400 pounds and those statistics were so frustrating. You know the ones:

"Statistically, most overweight people will never lose the weight."

"The average obesity rate in America is over 35 percent and rising drastically every year."

"A team of researchers at King's College found that only 1 in 220 men will lose their weight. And, if he's severely obese, he only has a 1 in 1290 chance of getting to a normal body."

"Higher risk of heart disease, heart attack, stroke..."

Blah, blah, blaaaaaaaah. These are all things you've heard a million times. I know I have. They are facts you know... well, maybe you can't say the cold, hard numbers, but deep down you *know* them.

The facts go in one ear and out the other. Why? There are a lot of reasons: Because they're all stating what we already know—being overweight is bad (Okay... duh). Because our identity is rooted in our physical shape (There's the big guy! Bruce will eat anything!). Because we justify why we are overweight (It's genetics. I have a thyroid condition.).

But deep down, we push the truth away because it makes us feel bad. It makes us feel like crap. We know we are overweight, and no matter how many body acceptance campaigns there are, we are miserable because of it. Knowing we could die because of our weight doesn't inspire us to lose it. It simply scares us, so why would we think about that?

The facts also say that even if we try to lose weight, we probably won't succeed. And even if we do succeed, we will simply gain the weight back in the near future (Oh that's great! #sarcasm). Who would even attempt to lose weight with that kind of cheer squad in their head?

You know the cigarette commercials where they show the negative effects of smoking? The one where the man can barely speak because he's breathing through a tube in his neck? Or the ads showing a gnarly black tumor in the lungs of a smoker? All fear tactics. And all of them have been statistically proven not to work. A guy did a study to prove it and published his findings in the *New York Times*.

Fear tactics don't work. It's because none of these facts or diets or workouts deal with the heart of the issue: You are overweight because you're using food to cope with the difficult things in your life.

Oh, I can hear you all crying out! "Bruce, that's wrong! I have more fat genes than everyone else!" "Bruce! You're so insensitive to people who have actual conditions that make it impossible for them to lose the weight!" "Bruce, I do NOT suffer from emotional eating, I just have a hearty appetite!" Or, my personal favorite, "I have a slower metabolism!"

You can yell and defend all day long, but deep down—for some of you, *very* deep down—you know just as well as I do that you're making excuses and justifying a bad habit: You're eating because you think your life is falling apart or to cope with what you can't handle.

I can say this truth without flinching because I've been where you are, right there in the darkness and self-loathing. The funny, fat friend who was secretly dying inside. I weighed over 400 pounds. Fun-loving Bruce with a dark secret. Food was my only comfort. It was my addiction.

But I have good news. I found my way out of that pit of despair. I lost ALL the weight. And more importantly, I learned what it means to have integrity and how to overcome my demons.

I was on ABC's *Extreme Weight Loss* and lost over 200 pounds. To say it changed my life is so cliché, but it's true. I wouldn't be the man I am today without what I went through and learned on that show. It was the hardest year of my life. I had to face a demon that to many, including myself, seemed unimaginable.

I'm not here to scare you. I'm not here to scold you. After going through the process, all I want in this whole world is to help you. I would rather die than not pass on what I learned. It sounds extreme, but it's true.

Now I know it's all about dealing with your heart. You've got to have a healthy spirit before you can even think about jumping on a treadmill. You've got fill up your love tank until it overflows before you start axing cookies from your life. You've got know that everything will be okay before you can start living a fulfilling life.

Because it's not about losing weight to make yourself healthy. It's about knowing you're capable of loving yourself, which will lead to loving others. That will make you the healthiest of all.

I have some pretty awful demons in my past. But I'm going to tell you how I overcame them. How I conquered something so evil it will make you sick.

Look, if I can do it, you can do it too. I beat the odds. I won't be labeled as a statistic. And you don't have to be either. It'll be hard. It sucks. But in the end, it's totally worth it!

I love to get pumped. So get pumped! This is it, people. This is the start of the rest of your life. Let's do this!

Chapter 1

Dad

I used to be over 400 pounds and I lost all the weight on ABC's *Extreme Weight Loss*. That's the story everyone knows. Where my story actually begins is with my dad and me. I loved my dad. He was my hero. If you were looking to have fun, Danny Pitcher was the guy to call. I looked up to him like no other, and I felt special that I got to spend almost all of my free time with him. It wouldn't be until later that I realized why he favored me so much. But I'm getting ahead of myself. Let's start at the beginning...

I was born in Provo, Utah. Go Utes! (Although in Provo, most people are BYU fans.) Like all of Utah, the majority of the town are members of the Church of Jesus Christ of Latter Day Saints (LDS). They are the friendliest and kindest people you'll ever meet.

My mom, Janet, suffered many miscarriages before me and had kind of given up on the idea of having children. Then BOOM! I came into the world and blessed everyone with my presence... Nah, I'm just kidding.

I was a normal-sized baby: 7 pounds, something ounces. So what happened? How did I go from under 10 pounds to over 400 pounds? That's a question that took me nearly my whole life to answer.

The thing about gaining a ton of extra, unwanted weight is that it usually starts before we even realize it. Gaining weight begins before we put on a single pound. Somewhere in our life, this little seed of darkness is planted in our psyche and then it grows and grows until we are overweight. Sometimes it's hard to see what the trauma might have been. It wasn't until I looked back that I realized my trauma was pretty easy to spot. So let's get back to my childhood.

My mom wasn't ever able to have any more biological children. But when I was five, I got a brother, Brandon. My parents adopted him as a baby. Apparently, I used to call Brandon *my* baby. I don't remember doing that, but I know for sure that I was excited to have a playmate. Today, towering over me, standing at 7 feet tall, Brandon is obviously not blood, but he is my family, and I went to great lengths to protect him.

My dad was super outgoing. This guy was beloved by our town. He was a football coach, a little league coach, a bus driver, and an all-around dynamic dude. For a guy who loved all things sports, he was actually incredibly artistic and was talented at it too. He was involved in local plays and musicals. He even sang in the church choir. This guy was doing all things at all times.

His creative side really shone during the holidays. He loved holidays, but especially Christmas. Every year our town would have a Christmas decoration contest and every year our house would win! My dad used to make wood cutouts of different things like the Nativity, the Peanuts gang, Looney Toons, or Santa and his reindeer. He painted them and put them in the yard with loads of other lights and Christmas decorations. It was the best.

It didn't stop on the inside of our house either. He would set up this giant train set that went around the whole living room. At night, he would tell Christmas stories as we sat in our little winter wonderland.

During the month of December, my dad, Coach Pitcher, would go the extra mile for his players. He used to go to each of his player's houses and hand-deliver Christmas cards. Since he never went anywhere without me, I got to ride along too! When he was working driving the bus, I would dress up like Santa and ride on the bus with him. We passed out candy canes and made everyone's day. We were a team.

But he didn't just do Christmas big. He did all holidays big: Thanksgiving, Fourth of July, every single holiday. My birthday is July 1, so we would always go to this big event for the Fourth and celebrate my birthday. When I was really little, I used to think the fireworks were just for me. My dad had a way of making you feel special. For the players on the teams he coached, he would celebrate their birthdays as well. He would invite the player over and make his famous chocolate malt milkshake for them. We would drink the milkshakes and have a great time. The parents trusted him because he was always going above and beyond to make sure the kids were safe. He would be the last one to leave the football field after a game. He made sure every player had a ride home—that every kid was taken care of.

All the players loved Coach Pitcher, so it meant that I had a lot of friends because they all liked my dad so much. They were always telling me things like, "Oh, your dad is just the man. He's the best dad ever." I used to think all the time, "Wow, I DO have the best dad ever, so I should be the best son ever and live up to those expectations of what a son of Dan Pitcher should look like."

Everything about my childhood felt perfect and magical. But what my innocent heart couldn't see was the trail of breadcrumbs my dad was already leaving behind. None of us could see it until we looked back. I didn't know that my parents had moved twice before landing in Provo. I didn't hear that both times they had to pack up and leave suddenly. I didn't know why my dad lost his teaching license. I didn't know there were events already set in motion that would alter my life forever.

People have different smarts. Some are street smart, some are book smart. I'm definitely not that last one. I'm people smart. I'm heart smart. But something I learned in school does stick in my memory: Newton's first law of motion. Weird, right? All it says is that something that is in motion will stay in motion. Well, I think about it because my dad was in motion—he was moving, sneaking around before I was even born. Then, when I came along, I was put in the path of that motion without even realizing it. The events in my life appeared to be already determined, the odds stacked against me.

Here's the thing, though, Newton's law doesn't just apply to my life, it applies to yours as well. There are things that were already in motion for your life too. We are all given a life with so many preset factors that we have no control over. It takes a long time to look back and see all the events that shape us. It takes a lot of work sometimes to recognize that things in play cause us to have a lot of baggage.

We all come with baggage. We all have things in our past that can affect our present and even our future if we allow them to. If you're reading this book, your baggage may be obvious: It may be your weight. But it may be something else too.

It doesn't feel great to look at the awful stuff that caused me to stumble. It doesn't feel great to know that I had no way of changing a lot of things. But it's important to look at those things. Whether I realized it or not, I ate food to comfort myself through all the bad times.

But once you're able to understand that we were all thrown into motion—a juggernaut—you're able to deal with it. Once you know you've got unwanted baggage tied to your back like a pack mule, you can overcome it. Once you pinpoint it and name it, you will find that you can have complete control over it. It won't be able to own you anymore. But it takes time and it takes integrity.

Take comfort in the fact that we were all thrown into a world where things were already in motion. We are all in this club together.

You can see the bags holding you down. Now you can begin to take them off, kick them to the curb, and take the first steps toward a new you.

I LIKE TO SAY TO MYSELF

I have baggage but life moves on.

Chapter 2

The Catalyst

When I was in second grade, I didn't have a care in the world. I liked watching *Teenage Mutant Ninja Turtles*. The only worry I had was that I wanted to be Michelangelo for Halloween, but my mom and I couldn't find the right shade of orange, so I settled on Leonardo because blue was easier to track down. I had that haircut where you take a bowl and put it on the top of your head and just cut. I was still a normal weight, not that I even thought about weight in second grade. I don't remember a whole lot from that year. But I do remember the helper who would sit next to me and some other kids in the classroom to make sure we understood everything. I would have a helper for almost all of my academic life. I didn't really mind, though. I always figured my helper was there to do exactly that: help. I walked to school, if you could even say that. Joaquin Elementary School was located directly across the street from my house. I can remember almost every teacher I ever had. Third grade was Mr. Branson. Fifth grade was Mrs. Whittingham. But the weird thing is that there is only one grade I can't recall who my teacher was: Second grade is the exception. For the life of me, I can't remember.

I think I have such trouble remembering that year because I was in second grade—I was eight years old—when the catalyst that would change the course of my entire life would occur. It was in that year that my dad started sexually molesting me. And he would continue to do so for six more years.

At the time, and for more than a decade after, I didn't think he was doing anything wrong. It took me a long time to realize it wasn't right.

How could I not know it was bad? Because my dad's abuse was all I'd ever known. Plus, my dad was the cookie-cutter definition of a child molester in that he conditioned me to think it was okay.

One of the saddest truths is that I wasn't his only victim. There were boys before me, boys throughout the six years I went through it. He had a type. They were always eight to fourteen years old. Those boys would prove to be braver than I was. They would be the ones to step forward when I shrank back. Those boys would be the reason he went to prison, not me.

There's a little story, I don't know where it came from, or who said it originally, but it goes like this: You can put a frog in a pot of water at room temperature and he won't mind. In fact, being an aquatic, amphibian creature, he will probably love it. If you turn on the heat and warm up the water just slightly, the frog won't notice. The water temperature is not that much different from when he was first placed in the pot to begin with. So you turn up the heat a little more. Again, it's a fine temperature to live in, so the frog is unaware. You can slowly keep raising the heat. After a certain point, it's hot in that pot, but the frog doesn't think about it because the whole process is so gradual. You can turn up the heat until eventually the pot of water is boiling. But the frog won't jump out. It will simply die. If you threw a frog in a pot of boiling water, he would jump out; but because you tempered and conditioned the frog first, he was unaware of how dangerous the situation was for him. And it cost him his life.

I was the frog, along with the other boys, and my dad was in control of the heat. His grooming process was almost identical to the frog in the pot. And just like the frog, our lives would be taken from us as well.

He was a master manipulator. He had a vetting process—a grooming method—to lure in victims. In the beginning, he would start out with something "innocent." Like, he would play a PG-13 movie with a sex scene, but nothing too graphic. Then he would ask the boy what he thought about it. Little stuff like that. If he got a "good" response, he would turn up the heat just a little, hotter and hotter. If at any point the victim started to push back, or he felt it wouldn't go well, he would abandon him and move on to another. Talking turned into light touches, which turned into a lot more. Before any of us realized it, we were in hot water, boiling away.

This whole process of turning up the heat was the real excitement for my dad. It's a classic characteristic for a molester. I think he got more satisfaction out of the process than the actual sexual acts.

My bedroom was in the basement of our little house. Just off to the side was another little room. We called it my dad's office, but really it was his lair to ruin someone's life. When I was eight, I found magazines that had been delivered to the house. Later, I would realize that my dad subscribed intentionally so I would find them. It wasn't anything too bad, not hard-core pornography. But they had scantily clad women on the cover and throughout. I took one down to my room and looked through it. Pictures like that spark curiosity within any boy that age. And with that curiosity comes guilt. The magazine stirred up a lot of feelings for a little boy like me. I will never forget my dad's voice when he caught me looking at it. It's still hard for me to talk about. "What are you looking at there, Bruce?" He wasn't angry. He was calm and acted as if it were the most normal thing in the world. His relaxed attitude made my guilt fade away. We began talking about all of the physical feelings those half-naked women were inspiring in me. He continued to tell me that all of that was natural. He continued to put me at ease.

That conversation was the catalyst—the crack in the door—for the rest of my life. Because from that point, it sparked much more. It was the catalyst for my depression, my ability to push emotions down. And even though I didn't know it, it was the catalyst for my weight gain. It was the start of the years of abuse I would take from my dad.

The definition of a catalyst is a person or event that quickly causes change or action. My father was the person who caused the event. He was my catalyst. Usually, a big moment is a good thing. But in my case, and maybe in your case, the big moment was a tragedy.

But here's what I've realized through years of counseling and introspection: If I hadn't been abused, I wouldn't be able to share my story in hopes of helping others. Sexual abuse is one of the worst things ever. As a victim, you never truly get over it. You learn to grow from it. I don't wish it on anyone. However, I can recognize that my abuse was the catalyst for my depression, my weight gain, my weight loss, and ul-timately my new life. From the ashes of the catalyst, I was reborn. And you can be too.

You have the ability to use your catalyst for something good. But you probably can't see it right now. That idea sounds crazy. But believe me, I know it is possible to use the worst possible catalyst to change your life for the better and help someone else. You might not be able to see it that way yet. Hang in there. With enough work, you will be able to one day.

I LIKE TO SAY TO MYSELF

Your catalyst brought about some good stuff.

Chapter 3

Get Ready to Rumble

efore I was born, my dad got his master's degree in teaching and eventually became a teacher. I don't remember exactly how old I was, but at some point in my childhood, my dad stopped working as a teacher. The details are fuzzy, but I remember my parents arguing about it. Maybe they were arguing about something else, though. They argued all the time. Anyway, I do know there was a rumor that had circulated about my dad's behavior with a certain male student. (Maybe it was multiple students, I don't know.) No charges were brought against him, but whatever was said was enough to get him fired. My mom wanted to know what that was all about. My dad quickly calmed her.

My dad always had a way of twisting things to make him come out good in the end. When he talked to you, you always felt like he was telling the truth. Now I can see that he was just really great at making up stories. Lying was as easy and effortless as breathing to my dad.

He told my mom she had it all wrong. He wasn't fired. He was simply moving on to a new career opportunity... as a bus driver. It was his choice. And as far as his accuser was concerned, obviously he was making it up. I didn't think much of any of it at the time. Hindsight is 20/20.

I also didn't think much about my parents' schedules either. My mom had a good job. She was working nights managing an office. My dad would get home from working for UTA (Utah Transit Authority) in the evening, around the time she was leaving for work. She would work all night and get home in time to get us ready for school in the morning. We would head off to school, my dad would go to work, and my mom would finally go to bed. My mom and dad lived on completely opposite schedules. During the week, they barely saw each other. On the weekends, my mom would forgo sleep so we could all be together.

Thinking about it now, this schedule suited my dad perfectly. With my mom gone at night, it was almost too easy for him to play out his sick life behind closed doors. I didn't know any of this, of course. That life was the only life I had known.

My dad asked me to tag along with him everywhere. I was always striving for my dad's love, so I loved that he wanted me around. I loved it most of the time. But sometimes it got to be a little too much. For instance, sometimes he would have me sit on the bus with him for his whole shift. That was pretty boring. On Sundays he liked to go for walks in the park. He basically insisted on it. I saw my friends at school, but most of the time outside of school, I was with my dad because he didn't like me being away from him. He also really didn't like it if I spent the night at my friends' houses. He was mean about it too. He would say things like, "Why don't you want to spend time with me?" If I ever did spend the night at a friend's house, he would be cold toward me and give me the silent treatment for a few days. I couldn't figure out why. All I knew was that it made me feel bad.

Having friends over to our house was a completely different story, though. He was totally cool about that. He would even request I invite certain friends over, saying things like, "We haven't seen so-and-so for a while. Wouldn't that be fun to have him over?" I just thought, alright, that does sound like fun.

I never knew my dad was doing the same things to them as he was to me. But looking back, I can see it clearly, and it makes me shudder. Here's a typical scenario that would happen when friends would come over: We would all go down to my basement room and hang out. My dad would come down and we would all watch a movie. It would be something seemingly innocent, like *Braveheart*. So, for instance, in the movie *Braveheart* there is a sex scene, nothing too graphic, though, so it didn't seem like anything was up. After the movie was over, my dad would talk to my friend about the movie. Then he would usually bring up the sex scene in a weird way. He would apologize for it, "I'm sorry you had to see that." But being apologetic brought sex into the conversation. It opened the door to that subject. It was all so subtle and manipulative that my friend wouldn't really realize that soon we were all talking and even joking about taboo subjects. He had a masterful way of disarming his victims and quieting any warning alarms that might go off in their head. Then my dad would find a way to get the boy in his office, next to my room. There would be something funny he had to show him. Something enticing that would peak his interest. Once he got him in there he would continue joking around about things most parents wouldn't joke around about. He would bring up masturbation, but in a casual, nonchalant way, like it was no big deal. Like I said before, if that went well, he would push it further. It would always be pretty late at this point, so I was usually falling asleep watching something. If the boy didn't spend the night, my dad would drive him home. I can still hear his voice as I was trailing off, "Bruce, I'm going to take him home." I don't like thinking about what happened to my friends on those car rides. I feel too much guilt.

I don't remember exactly how old I was, but around middle school, my family began fostering kids. This will make you sick. They weren't just any kids; my dad requested boys, ages eleven to fourteen. Just like with my friends, I never once thought that my dad was talking to them, touching them, sodomizing them, and destroying their lives. My dad had the perfect set up. He had a large pool to draw from—an endless supply for an endless appetite. I hate thinking about it now.

That was my life, though. That was my truth. It took me years to learn that all of it was a lie. A strange side effect after I learned the truth is that now I'm embarrassed by all of it. My dad's behavior—that seemed so normal at the time—makes me uncomfortable now. It sounds weird, but it's almost like I had to learn to feel bad about something that I thought was good. This is all compounded by the fact that my dad repeatedly coached me and drilled me not to say anything. I want to share my story now. But I have to admit, there's still a part of me that has trouble doing that. I know it wasn't my fault. It took me years to understand that my dad's actions were evil. Yet, when I write these things about my dad, there's still a small part of me that feels guilty for doing so. There's still a part of me that wants to protect him. The monster in him groomed me to be his shield. My life was so intertwined with his that I had to defend both of us.

And that's what I will always have to fight against. When battling your own demons, you fight them and they go away, but they'll come back. We all end up fighting the same demons over and over again. That's a part of life. It's also a big part of growth and building your integrity. The more tools you acquire, the more times you fight, the easier it becomes. I have to work hard not to feel like my father's protector. I have to work even harder not to blame myself. But with every victory, I receive new life. I get pumped.

I LIKE TO SAY TO MYSELF

It may be the same demon, but you're fighting it well today.

Chapter 4

Life Lessons of Football

I did inherit something from my dad that is pure and innocent, untainted by his abuse: a love for football and all things sports. Football has and always will be one of the biggest parts of my life. I love it, man. I love watching the games, studying the playbook, and getting on the field throwing around the pigskin. Football helped me escape. Because it's not about winning or losing. It's a team sport. The greatest team sport in all of sports. Yeah, it's great to wake up on the weekends and watch the games. But there's something bigger behind it. There's a family behind it.

For all you non-football peeps out there, I just want to let you know that a lot of my better qualities were developed through the sport. It teaches teamwork, responsibility, and loads of other things. But the thing I owe most to football is that it taught me to work hard and to love and support others.

I started playing football when I was twelve. My weight at this point was still fairly in check. I had baby fat and that usual pudginess that kids in middle school get. I didn't even think about my weight at that age.

During the day, my dad was my football coach. And at night, my dad would take me down to the basement, three to four nights a week, where we would take turns on each other. I was his favorite, after all. I still thought all of that was normal.

You would think that maybe as a coach he would show favoritism toward me. But my dad always had a strange (twisted, evil, demented) way of showing me "love." He was actually hardest on me during practices and games. He was downright brutal.

Before football, I played little league baseball. During one game, my dad got so angry that I was striking out that he went into a monster rage. He was screaming at me until he was red in the face. He looked like a wild animal. It was so bad that after the game, the police came to my house to make sure everything was okay. I knew how to protect my dad because he had already prepped me on what to say should something like this happen. He was never like, "Here's what to say if a policeman comes to the door." But he did explain how "special" our relationship was. He would beat around the bush when trying to secretly condition me to protect him. My dad would always talk to me about how, because our relationship was so special, no one would understand it because it was so great and unique. That's the argument he would use to get the idea into my psyche. I've already talked about how out in public he had this dazzling, outgoing personality that everyone loved and admired. No one would know anything different about Coach Pitcher because I was never alone with anyone to tell them. (It's not like I would've anyway.) There was so much positive energy surrounding my dad that I just felt extra special to be what felt like the apple of his eye. When people would go on and on about my dad, I would think, yeah, and little do they know I have such a great relationship with him. Everyone was so dazzled by him and loved him. I felt extra good because I had an even more intimate and close relationship that people didn't know about. It made me feel special that I had this secret with my dad... at least that's what my dad got me to think. So when the police came to our house that night after the game, after being verbally abused by him, I stood up for my dad and his "great" character and how he was a great dad.

But the verbal and psychological abuse under his coaching didn't let up. My football games weren't much better. I remember one time in seventh grade we had a big playoff game. Right before halftime, we were on the one-yard line about to start. We all huddled up. My dad called the play, and we ran out onto the field. But when I got out there, I forgot the snap count. It messed up everything. We were penalized. The other team continued to score the rest of the night.

We lost that night. All of us walked off of the field feeling super dejected. We lost because of a bunch of collective mistakes we made together. But when we gathered around my dad, he singled me out and said to the whole team, "We lost tonight because of you, Bruce." I've never felt more humiliated in my entire life than when he called me out in front of everyone like that.

My dad never should've treated me like that. However, while I may have a knack for the coaching and strategy of the game, the truth is, I'm not very good at *playing* sports. I'm not bad. I'm mediocre. I love 'em, though. Throughout my time as a player, I had to work twice, three times as hard as everyone else. But I never gave up. When my dad would constantly tell me what a terrible player I was, I worked harder.

And I managed to get to a higher level. Not the highest, but the highest for me.

I can't say it enough, but even when my dad would lose it, I still thought he was the greatest. He used to tell me he was hard on me because he didn't want the other guys thinking he was showing favoritism. He always twisted all his bad behavior into something positive. "I'm hard on you because it's good for you." Which I translated to, "I'm hard on you because I love you, Bruce." But the truth, I can see so clearly now, is that my dad was just plain hard on me.

I was always eager to make my dad proud of me. So I worked like no other. It would be years down the road before I would learn that I was actually channeling the myth, the legend, my hero, Jerry Rice. This guy will go down in history as one of the greatest players in NFL history. I will expand on it later, but Jerry told me, "I think the thing about that was I was always willing to work; I was not the fastest or biggest player, but I was determined to be the best football player I could be on the football field, and I think I was able to accomplish that through hard work."

Like Jerry Rice, I wasn't naturally the best, but I got better through a ton of hard work. (I never quite got to the level of Jerry, though.) One good thing that came out of my dad putting so much pressure on me was that I learned how to work hard. Later, when I was on *Extreme Weight Loss*, I already knew how to kill a workout. Football practice planted a seed to teach me how to physically push myself, which was paramount in helping me lose weight.

Even at my heaviest, I still worked hard. Football taught me that. You don't have to be the best *person* in the world, you just have to be the best *you* in the world. Don't pine away for the star athlete (or person) you wish you could be. You can learn from the best, but spend that energy working on your own skills.

I LIKE TO SAY TO MYSELF

You're working so hard, Bruce!

Chapter 5

Janet

"He had such a hold on me," my mom says when she talks about her controlling husband, my dad, "He was so deceitful."

When you visit my mom's house, she will immediately apologize for the state of her living space. At first glance, her house appears to just be filled with clutter. But when you take a moment to really look, you can learn a lot about her. Most of the "mess" is made up of sewing projects. My mom was and still is a very talented seamstress. She made all of my costumes for Halloween, which always made me feel I had the best costumes, because I did. And she didn't stop there. My mom made costumes for the high school musicals, wedding attire, everyday clothes, and everything in between. But her home is comfortable and has a lived-in feel. While a lot of the things bring a lot of warmth and life, behind all the trinkets are remnants from a hellish life being married to my dad.

"We had so much fun when we first met," my mom says about that charismatic man that most people knew and loved. They went out all the time. To the public, my dad kept up his jubilant façade. "As a coach, he only wanted the very best for his players." My mom and I can remember how Coach Pitcher used to try and make all of us boys feel like we were in the NFL. He would get our names embroidered on our jerseys. "I made little towels with the logo and name decals for them to have in the locker room," my mom reminds me.

I felt special, the kids felt special, and the parents of the players were overjoyed by these "selfless" acts of kindness. But only my mom knew the real motivation behind everything, "He always had to look good. Everything was over-the-top and dramatic. It was all about him." Too true.

His demonstrative acts of attentiveness and kindness as a coach never seemed to make their way into the home he shared with us, though. "It was the most miserable time of my life when he taught football," my mom will say, with an unmistakable note of bitterness in her voice. "If he lost a football game Friday night, no one could even talk to him until Monday after football practice, otherwise he would bite your head off."

My dad's insatiable need for grandeur didn't stop with his players. He himself never wanted for anything. My mom slaved away, working nights, but immediately had to hand over her paychecks to my dad for him to spend how he pleased. "He thought, if it didn't cost the most, it wasn't the best to buy." My mom talks about the list of goodies my dad would bestow upon himself: big screen TVs, surround sound, a laser disc player. While my mom drove a beater car, my dad got himself a fancy Mazda Protégé in dark green. A smooth ride that my mom was never able to experience because my dad wouldn't allow her to drive his car.

Danny Pitcher would zip around town as a beloved coach, outgoing church member, and jolly bus driver. But behind closed doors, when he didn't have to worry how he looked to others, he was an out-of-control tyrant that dictated nearly every aspect of our family's life.

It wasn't always that way, according to my mom. When I was a baby, apparently my dad was a selfless and doting father. At the time, a cunningly intelligent Danny was working on his master's degree from BYU. "He was a loving father. He would help out and everything. Then he turned into this monster," my mom recalls.

Just like what I've said, my dad seemed to put a spell on his victims, my mom included. We hated it. It was always uncomfortable at home and I always had a knot in my stomach when my dad would spin his tales. "He always had a story that made sense." My mom struggled with the allegations that were brought up throughout their marriage, the whispers in the towns they fled. There were rumors and signs that his pedophilia began before my parents even met. A classic trait of pedophiles is that they always have it on their minds. It's always a part of their plan. However, no plan is airtight. So if my mom ever asked him about something bad, my dad always had a way of talking her down from any assumptions. He was a master manipulator.

Blow-up fights and days of silence were a way of life for my mom. Love and affection became nonexistent. But instead of leaving the situation, my mom was determined to stay with him for Brandon and me. "I was raised to think that no matter how hard things got, you keep your family together. It's a forever family." It's difficult to look back and see that staying for us kids might actually have been a bad thing. But I've never blamed my mom for anything that happened to me, or to the family. She was a victim too.

Under the stress of it all, my mom gained a lot of weight—around 200 pounds to be exact. Years later, after my dad went to prison, he spun a story in front of his sister, his parents, and my mom. He always maintained that he was "mostly" innocent. But as for any little acts of indiscretion, he blamed my mom: It was because my mom was so repulsively fat that he had to get intimacy from somewhere else. Because my mom gained weight, he was no longer attracted to her and had to sodomize little boys. Somehow, and tragically, his family thought this sounded like a valid argument. But the more you hear about him, the more you understand that his spellbinding, storytelling abilities seem to sink in deep. He hypnotized not just his family but every person he met as well.

My mom will begin tearing up from the crippling guilt she feels for me and the other victims. I always try to comfort her and let her know it's not her fault. I'll say, "Mom, it's not your fault. Always know that I love you with all my heart and would not be the man I am today without you." She is usually inconsolable. She wracks her brain every day, trying to understand how she missed all the signs. But when my mom got the call from my dad that he had been arrested, she felt completely blindsided. And I know she's telling the truth.

For years, my mom has had to live with the agony of wondering how, as a mother, she could've done better. She did her best to push down those feelings and move on with her life. But when I was chosen for the show, all of that guilt was brought to the forefront.

My mom is quick to praise ABC's *Extreme Weight Loss*. She feels forever indebted to all the people who were a part of it: "The show saved us." But she adds, "When they came to film, I was so nervous to have the producers grill me." They asked her a series of questions that are readily on anyone's mind when they hear my story: "You were the mother, how could you not know?" "Where were you?" "Did you turn a blind eye?" "You had to know something was going on." My mom said that all of it made her question everything about herself: "The questions they asked made me think, what does that make me look like as a mother, that I didn't know?" She can never keep from crying when she thinks about it, "I punish myself every day because I didn't know. And what was I not seeing?"

But it's hard to see things when you're in them. Perspective is always gained by looking back. Now when my mom looks at her life and the life of our family, what seemed normal takes on a more sinister feel. "When I look back on the things, I can see clearly now. Like, I would always have Brandon with me, and he would always have Bruce with him. He never really ever left Bruce with me. But I didn't put two and two together on that because it was football practice and all those things. And then I was working and I had a really good job, but it was at nights." She never suspected that her husband could be molesting his own son.

With all the ups and downs, through everything that's happened, my mom has remained resilient and tough as nails. Free from the shackles of my dad, my mom is living a whole new life. She admits with tears of joy, "I think our family is receiving our blessings now." And she, just like me, is very passionate, and I love it.

Chapter 6

Impress Me

It would be a long time before my mom would be able to have that kind of clarity and understanding about what we all went through.

I never saw my parents be affectionate toward one another. No hugs. No holding hands. We would all be together, but the love wasn't there. And when I really look back, the love wasn't there between my dad and me either. I thought he loved me. But someone who loves you shouldn't constantly put you down. And that's exactly what my dad did.

I was never good enough, and my dad was quick to point it out. The truth is, no one is ever "good enough" in the sense that no one is perfect. My dad would constantly compare me to other kids—peers my age—and tell me I needed to be like them. He would point out a specific kid and say, "Why can't you be like so and so? Look what he does. This is why people like him. This is why he has so many friends. You should be like him." I think he was saying that so he would have control over me. All a kid wants in the whole world is his dad's approval and love. So when my dad put me down, I would always try to gain his admiration. It made for a relationship where I was always inferior, seeking my father's love. Mentally, it put me in a weak position, which was exactly where he wanted me. He beat me down emotionally so much that he could easily control me. I had no thoughts that were my own.

I still have to fight against my dad's voice in my head. I used to hear my dad's voice in my head a thousand times a day, telling me that I needed to be impressive. I wanted to be special to my dad. I wanted him to talk about me like he talked about the other players—how they did so many great things. I always thought, "Why can't I get to that point?" because it never seemed to happen for me.

Later, when I started *Extreme Weight Loss*, I finally got to a point where I said, "You know what? I did something amazing." I could do it. I started to see that I could be great, that I could be a motivator and a leader, and that I'm good enough.

To truly be able to believe that you're good enough, you have to not care what other people think of you. Part of integrity is knowing who you are and that who you are is good. My dad was holding me back when he was around, and long after he was gone, because I continued to care what he thought about me. All that worry and anxiety was channeled to my eating. I would feel inferior, which would make me eat and gain weight, making me feel even more inferior. It was a vicious cycle. What would your life be like if you didn't care what anyone thought about you? How would you act? Look inside yourself and find the truth about who you are. If you really look, you'll find that you are good. That's the truth, and it really does set you free.

I have to fight every day to live my truth. And you can too. Just because you've learned the truth doesn't mean everything will be easy. I actively block out my dad's voice. At first it was really hard. But it got easier and easier as time went on. There is a battle going on every day between good and evil. I must make the decision to listen to the good and mute the evil.

I LIKE TO SAY TO MYSELF

You're good enough.
You're good enough.
You're good enough.

Chapter 7

Gone

My whole life was turned upside down in one day. I remember it vividly. It was April 30, 1999. That was a Friday. I was fourteen and noticeably putting on weight at this point. It was first period PE, which started at 7:45 a.m. We were playing basketball inside because there was a chill in the air outside. I was wearing all white—white shorts, white shirt—the sacrificial lamb about to go to the alter. We hadn't been playing even a half hour before the coach called me over. He had a slip in his hand requesting I go to the office.

I walked down the hall, having no idea why I was summoned. I wasn't anxious or worried. It felt routine.

When I got to the office, the receptionist greeted me. She called in the back and a sheriff appeared. He was friendly. He shook my hand and asked if I would take a ride with him. I still had no idea what was going on, but I said, "Sure."

Still in my PE clothes, I walked out of the school, and I got in his cop car. During the drive, the sheriff just asked me how school was going, how was the football season, etc. I didn't have the slightest clue why I was in the car. I thought I was just on this special ride. There was a big campaign going on for cops at the time. I thought it was a buddy system thing. Or maybe a "Be a Cop for a Day" thing. We drove down to south Provo, into a normal neighborhood. There were little houses along the road, nothing out of the ordinary.

We pulled up to a house with a green door and green trim around the windows. The only weird thing was this house had a parking lot and no yard. I didn't know who lived there. When we got inside, the layout was like a normal house, but the furniture wasn't quite right.

They took me to a bedroom, but there were no beds in it. It had a green couch, a little white table, and some plastic chairs in it. There were teddy bears in the corner, with one really big white teddy bear. It caught my eye for some reason. I found out later that this was a forensics house used for interviewing potential victims of child sexual abuse. But at the time, I didn't know that, and I was beginning to feel a little anxious. I thought maybe I was in trouble for some stupid stuff I had done with my friends. Did we break something over the weekend? Were we making too much noise at Corey's house? The thought that it could be something involving my dad never even entered my head.

The sheriff pulled up a chair and placed a tape recorder on the table. I wracked my brain trying to think what I had done wrong. What was I in trouble for? The first question he asked me was, "How is your relationship with your dad?" Then I knew exactly why I was there. I became numb and immediately went into defense mode. My dad warned me about something like this happening. He had prepped me for years in advance to say nothing. My dad's words were rattling in my head, "These people will try to take you away from me. What would you do if I weren't in your life? Could you imagine? You wouldn't make it." All I could think of was protecting my dad and keeping him out of jail, because he had convinced me that I needed him to survive.

The questions kept coming, "Has your dad ever touched you inappropriately?" It took me a little too long to answer. I was in shock. Then I told the lie I would continue to tell for over six more years: "No." I had never told anyone about what had been going on for the past six years. And I wasn't about to now. I denied everything. I would save my dad because I loved my dad. I thought I *needed* my dad.

I thought I had done a good job of saying nothing, but looking back, I know they knew. It was written all over my face and in my body language. But without an admission, they couldn't do anything. So they took me back to school.

On the ride back to school, the sheriff was trying to be really kind. He was asking me normal questions because he could tell I was just anxious as could be.

The first thing I did was go back to the office and call my mom. I said, "Mom, the police just came and took me." She said, "I know. The police just came and took your dad."

When I think about it now, I think about how messed up it was. My dad was my abuser, yet I wanted to look out for him, when it should've been the exact opposite. I denied everything and said my dad never made me watch porn and never let me go to a sleepover because he wanted me that night. I didn't think about how he always kept me by his side so I wouldn't have the opportunity to tell someone something. I just pushed it from my mind, like I always had. I went home that night, and my dad was gone. But my problems were just beginning.

Chapter 8

Can I Get a Ride, Coach?

My dad came from a big family. Who are we kidding? Most families are big in Utah. He had three older brothers and one older sister. There was a large age gap between my dad and his siblings. He was a surprise baby who came a lot later. I don't know if my grandparents fed him with an actual silver spoon, but my dad was definitely spoiled. His parents had a lot of land in Logan, Utah, and the surrounding area. They sat on quite a little fortune.

When my dad was arrested, his bail was set at $25,000. One phone call to his parents, and my dad made bail. Not wanting to lose the $2,500 down payment, they didn't go through a bail bondsman either. Without batting an eye, they simply wrote a check for the lump sum because they had the money and much more to spare.

After my dad was arrested, and then made bail, our little town of Provo was a media circus. The entire state of Utah tuned in. We had reporters camped outside our house for weeks. Living across from an elementary school made things even worse. News outlets would interview parents dropping their kids off at school, asking what they thought about a sexual predator lurking just across the street. And you guessed it: People were sickened. The negative press never seemed to stop, either. At the end of the year, it was the number one news story for the entire year. My dad's mug shot was on the six o'clock news every night.

The hardest part for me was that I missed my dad. I know that sounds weird, but I can't stress enough that I didn't understand that what he did was wrong. I missed watching games with him and going on drives with him. But I also missed having what I thought was a "normal" life. I started putting on more weight than I should've at this point because I was using food as a coping mechanism. It was obvious to everyone around me now that I was overweight.

When he came back home after making bail, the sexual abuse stopped entirely. The whole focus became how are we going to get Dad out of this one? What can we do to show everyone that he is innocent? My dad kept telling us that everyone was watching our every move, so it was very important to look like a loving family. There was so much pressure because, according to him, if we didn't, he would go to prison. He would say things like, "Is that what you want? For me to be gone forever?" He would always emphasize how bad off we would be if he weren't in our lives.

At home my dad maintained his innocence, but out in the world, everyone was telling me that everything I had known was a lie. I thought my dad loved me more than anyone else, yet everyone was screaming at me that he didn't love me *at all.* Not at all? I couldn't wrap my head around that. I thought my dad was the greatest guy in the world, but now everyone was saying that he was a sick, demented, horrible human, not worthy to even live. I thought my dad cared about me, but journalists were saying he harmed me. Well, technically they weren't saying he harmed *me*, because at that point no one knew he had touched me. While the police suspected he had abused me, they couldn't prove it. So everyone innocently thought I had only been hurt by his actions against others.

I don't mean to play the "poor me" card, but I have to set the scene a little. My mom's life was falling apart too. She was getting a lot of heat because how could she not know what he was up to? My dad and mom blamed me for my dad being in prison, even though that makes no sense at all. And on top of everything else, I had some pretty bad bullies at my school. I was on the football team (of course), and I had a lot of trouble with some of the other players at first.

Shortly after my dad went to prison, I went back to the locker room to get my backpack after practice. Other players were around. I could hear them snickering, but I didn't think much of it. I had to open my backpack to put something in it and saw something completely disgusting and humiliating. Someone had defecated in it. I can't describe what that felt like. The only thing I remember was being frozen from shock. Like, I just couldn't process it. When I think about it now, I know they were just immature guys messing around. A couple of bad eggs who didn't understand the situation. But at the time I just felt super depressed. That was one of the worst years of my life.

But in that year, I would form bonds and relationships with real men. Men who would become my father figures. Men who would teach me and fill in all the areas my dad had neglected. These men were my coaches. My dad took advantage of boys because, as their coach, he was in a position of guidance, leadership, and—most importantly—power. But my coaches showed me what a coach should look like. They demonstrated how to properly interact with and treat their players, and how to use that power for good.

Sometimes it's hard to see any good in a bad situation. But my coaches were the good for me. I always get choked up when I think about what they've done for me. Always take a look and locate the people who truly care about you. They're out there.

I LIKE TO SAY TO MYSELF

This sucks, but there's always something good.

Chapter 9

Bravery

I think the biggest surprise for people when they hear my story is the fact that I've never made any accusations against my dad. I did not help get him arrested in any way. It was the opposite. I did everything I could and said everything I "should" so he would not go to jail. My efforts proved to be unhelpful. Thankfully, the truth always comes out.

It all started when a group of players were hanging out at one of their houses. I wasn't there, so the details are fuzzy. My dad was a coach and had been grooming and molesting his players for years. Like me, all of them were quiet about it. Then one day a kid mentioned something casually about how Coach Pitcher had said and done some weird things. It was probably something about how my dad would find a way to bring up sexual, off-limits subjects. Or how he would touch them, in a casual, benign way, but it felt like more. As soon as the kid said that, many more guys started chiming in with their own similar stories involving Coach Pitcher. All the guys got to talking. Their conversation was overheard by a parent who was concerned by what he heard and decided to investigate.

Many kids came out of the woodwork, but it was only two victims who actually pursued legal justice. After all of the depositions, my dad had twenty-two charges brought against him, including three counts of sodomy on a child, five counts of sexual abuse on a child, and over ten counts of forcible sexual abuse on a child—which are all felonies—and multiple other misdemeanors. The boys were thirteen years old.

At first, my dad pled not guilty to all counts. However, the case never went to trial because his lawyers told him his best shot was to take a plea deal. So my dad admitted to two acts of sodomy on a child, hopeful that he would get less prison time than if he tried to battle out the twenty-two counts in court. The other twenty counts were dropped. The judge gave him the maximum sentence of fifteen years to life. My dad was floored. We were all floored.

I never testified because they never knew I had been abused the worst of all. To this day, I haven't sought any legal action against my dad. This is hard for me to cope with now. The bravery those victims had is incredible. They possessed something I didn't at the time. Because they stepped forward, many other potential victims have been spared.

I was blinded by a false love for my dad. When I decided to protect him, instead of to prosecute him, it wasn't the right thing to do. I learned the hard way that there is incredible strength in standing up for yourself. But don't learn it like I learned it. You can be brave right now. You can look your adversity in the face and defeat it.

I LIKE TO SAY TO MYSELF

You are brave.

Chapter 10

Coach Wong and Coach Clark

"He had a love for football. I think he got it from his dad," Coach Wong begins. Wong is a former offensive lineman from Hawaii, and to say he is a big guy is an understatement. He is a giant teddy bear with a relaxed, island attitude.

Coach Wong began coaching Bruce in his junior year, after his dad had gone to prison. "There was something peculiar about him. He wasn't your typical football athlete. There seemed to be a darker side. I didn't know what it was at the time." Coach Wong did what he says he did for all the athletes: He got to know them on a personal level. He, along with the other coaches, figured out Bruce's strengths and weaknesses. "As we got to know Bruce better we knew there were some situational things, financial challenges. Not super book-smart, but what we did know about Bruce was that if we challenged him and pushed him, he would rise to the occasion."

Coach Wong describes Bruce in high school as a withdrawn teen with very low confidence. Eventually, Wong discovered the truth about his father. Things made more sense after that. Even though it would be many more years before

Bruce would confess that his father sexually molested him, Wong said, "I knew he had. Just based on behavior, I knew he had been. Because that's normally where it starts. Bruce would misbehave. Also, clinging to us was a sign. He was always around us, even outside of school. Whenever something negative would happen, I had a feeling that he definitely had been abused."

"In the beginning, I had no idea either. I always kind of wondered," Coach Clark chimes in, "Then I heard some stories and I thought, poor guy. There's problems with his dad." Coach Clark is also a Hawaii native. He has a slow way of speaking that is calm, yet assertive. With eight kids of his own, Clark is the ultimate father figure to Bruce. "My wife said, what happened to all your money? I would tell her, 'Well Bruce is around, what do you think?'" Both Wong and Clark laugh as they remember how Bruce was always "forgetting" his wallet.

Bruce hung around his coaches outside of school. He would go over to their houses for football games on Sunday. He would go out to eat with them. One thing everyone agreed on is that Bruce did not share food!

That year the pieces of Bruce's life had been completely scattered. He never had consistency. But these men were there for Bruce when his real father wasn't. They guided him and helped him become the man he is today. They brought structure to his life. But most important, they brought love, shown in many different ways. They helped him in school, at home, in everyday activities. They helped Bruce with his car troubles. He almost always needed a ride. They helped him move. "How many times did Bruce help me move?" Coach Clark says with a smile, "None!" Although Bruce swears he helped for "at least an hour."

Chapter 11

One Big, Happy Family
in Prison

My coaches were slowly filling in the father-figure-sized hole I had. But all their love didn't keep me from having to see my dad in prison.

After his conviction, my dad's battle wasn't over. In his mind, and probably in ours as well, he was still going to get out. My parents stayed married. So throughout my remaining high school years, everyone was determined to help right a wrong that had been done to my dad.

Even though I already wanted to see my dad, it was weird because he also demanded I visit him in prison. He basically forced my mom and Brandon to visit as well. So we would go see my dad at least twice a week. Every visit was the same—how were we going to get dad out of here? He was so particular about us visiting because he thought it made him look good. With his family standing by him, he would look like the innocent man he was and get out early.

During a lot of the visits, my eyes would just glaze over as he shared the same ideas over and over again. I know now that it was a coping mechanism for me. That's the only way I can figure it. Because he would go on and on about how all the kids who stepped forward were lying, when I knew they weren't. I had experienced, firsthand, all the charges brought against him by other kids. Yet I didn't flinch or get upset when my dad sat across from me and told anyone who would listen that he was innocent. I think I also subconsciously justified his behavior. Since it was all I knew, I didn't view it as bad, so why would he go to prison for it?

Plus, if we didn't see him, boy, was he mad. He would be so mean. In his mind, if we missed even one potential visit, he would be locked away forever. There was insane pressure on us to get him out. I hated that. But we didn't want to anger him, and we did want him to get out, so we planned our lives around prison visits. We missed out on so many things because we went to see him. We would skip weekends, holidays, and big events so we could visit my dad in prison. At the time, we were determined to stand by him. We were still gripped by his manipulative hand.

He also called home almost every night. As much as he and my mom didn't get along, he wanted her to talk to him. Calls from prison are expensive. My mom was paying hundreds of dollars a month just so my dad could talk to her about how miserable he was.

What we did to see and talk to my dad went on for years—all through high school and even after. Looking back, seeing my dad had some nice moments, but it didn't bring me any joy. It was slowly killing me, and I couldn't recognize it. My brother, Brandon, did. He would often skip out on visits. He had more clarity than Mom or me. I think it was because he didn't suffer as much abuse. He says my dad never sexually molested him. I believe him because, for one thing,

Brandon was just a little too young. My dad didn't typically start with boys until they were at least eight or nine. (Brandon was eight when my dad was arrested.) And also, sadly, I don't think my dad paid much attention to Brandon because he was adopted. Brandon was always with my mom, and I was always with my dad. That's just how it was.

We all coped in different ways. Brandon simply says he doesn't remember any of it. But a therapist told me Brandon probably has just locked it far away in his mind and that it will take a long time to get out. I coped by eating. I was eating fast food all the time. The physical activity of football was the only thing keeping me from going over 300 pounds. But no matter how you slice it, this was a difficult time in my life. I had to relearn what normal was. But all I ended up doing was becoming numb. I pushed everything down in this phase and decided I just wouldn't deal with it. But what gets pushed down comes out eventually. If I have any advice, it's this: Don't become numb to things. Allow yourself to go through it. Because when you push things down, you begin carrying the baggage without even knowing it.

I LIKE TO SAY TO MYSELF

You won't feel full by pushing things down.
You'll only feel empty.

Chapter 12

Toughness

After my dad was arrested, I wasn't the only one whose world was crumbling around them. Brandon's life was turned upside down too. But the person it affected most of all was my mom, Janet.

She had endured her own type of abuse from my dad. He was controlling every part of her life. And he was mean about it. Most of the time, my mom would be stoic and just let him, but other times she would fight him. Their fights were explosive—screaming and yelling. After the storm came the silence. They wouldn't speak to each other for weeks at a time.

He would belittle my mom. He forced her to work and be gone from the house. All of his behavior makes sense, looking back at it now. He didn't want her home because he wanted the house empty to carry out his devilish activities. But at the time, he was making my mom's life a living hell.

He had a way he wanted us to do everything. From how to keep the house, to how and when we would go on vacation.

We used to go to his parents' house for Thanksgiving. My grandparents didn't get along with my mom. On those visits, it wasn't just my dad against my mom, it was my dad and his parents ganging up on her. There would be fighting, and then she would usually spend the rest of the time in her room.

But through everything, she stayed with my dad. Both my parents were a part of the LDS church, and both felt divorce wasn't an option. She stuck it out and did the best she could.

From the day they came and took my dad away, my mom's life was altered forever. People suspected I had been abused, which didn't feel great. But they suspected my mom knew what my dad was up to for all those years, which is much worse. They labeled Brandon and me as victims, but they labeled my mom as a negligent mother—a co-conspirator with my dad because she "let" him continue his abuse. Everyone had the same thought about her, "How could she not know?"

My mom didn't know. I can say this with certainty because I was there. I think the hardest thing for people to understand about my dad is that he is a master manipulator. He is shrewd and cunning. He is brilliant at twisting things in a way that always has him coming out looking like a good guy. Living in a home with him has an intoxicating effect, and not in a good way. His controlling and manipulative behavior causes you to be under his spell. You can't see clearly. You can't think clearly. You're not living in the real world. You're living in Danny Pitcher's world. Like a snake charmer, he plays his flute, and you dance for him.

The only people who know what it's like to be so deceived are Brandon, my mom, and me. She didn't know the horrors that were taking place in her own home, night after night, year after year, because my dad blinded her to it. He verbally beat her down to the point that she had to be numb to life just to survive.

My dad's spell continued to plague us even after he went to prison. He kept telling us he didn't do what they said. He blamed everyone else for why he was there.

But watching my mom go through all of this has given me great respect for her. Yeah, we have definitely had our struggles, but my mom is the toughest person I know.

When my dad went to prison, she had her moments where she was crying, and she had her down times. Everyone is allowed times in their life when they want to die. I like to use the analogy of a cancer patient. They fight and work to survive, but you can't expect them to always have a smile on their face. They need a few people they can cry to. They need an inner circle where they can just let their emotions out.

My mom was so tough around my brother and me. She rarely wavered. She found other people to cry to. But to us she would just say, "We're going to be okay. We're going to make it." From the moment my dad stopped working, money was always tight. But even when our power was shut off, or the water stopped running, my mom always managed to have food in the house and to get the bills paid as soon as she could.

That is what toughness is all about. It's about a person who battles adversity and takes it head on and keeps on moving.

There are so many moments over the years when my mom demonstrated to me what toughness looks like. But one story sticks out in particular.

After my dad went to prison, my mom decided to start her new life. She figured that started with losing weight. With the same shared abuse and horrors in our past, my mom and I gained weight for the same reasons. Like me, my mom was also 200 pounds overweight. When I was in high school, she had gastric bypass surgery. While that kind of surgery can have quicker results, it's by no means easier. You have to write down every meal, every gram of sodium, and log every ounce of water. You have to be extremely diligent. You have to go to countless doctor visits. You constantly have needles in your arm. After the operation, you feel sick. You can hardly keep anything down. You're just as hungry, but when you eat, it makes you nauseous. It's no walk in the park. But my mom got through it with flying colors.

After losing the fat, only the skin remains—so much skin. My mom then underwent skin surgery to have it removed. I remember her saying it was the most painful experience you could have, but it didn't register with me. Plus, she defied the odds and made it seem like it wasn't that bad. After the surgery, the doctors advise you to take it easy for four to six weeks—limited movement and bed rest. My mom, the toughest person I know, got out of bed after four days and went to work! I can't even fathom it. If that doesn't say tough, I don't know what does. She went back because she knew she had to provide for Brandon and me. She made sure we had money to put food on the table, pay for our utilities, fill the car with gas, and for all of the other things we needed.

Fast forward to more than a decade later when I finally became the new man I am today. It was after the show. My skin removal surgery was fast approaching, and I was super stoked. I affectionately referred to the belly skin pancake I had as Jerome. (No Jerome flapping around when I did my burpees!) I didn't even think about the fact that they would literally cut me in half—a perfect circle around my middle— pull down the skin from my abdominal wall, my sides, and my back, slice off the extra, and staple it all down with one hundred staples. My mom warned me about the physical pain this surgery would cause, but still I didn't really listen. She kept telling me to get ready because it would be horrific.

People can tell you something they learned from experience all day long, but for some of us simple people, until we experience it ourselves, we don't listen.

It took me about two seconds after the surgery to realize that my mom was 100 percent right. Holy crap. It was excruciating. I've never experienced pain like that before. Every movement hurt. Breathing hurt. Just sitting in my bed hurt. I'm telling you right now that I would rather jump in a pool of salt water with a bunch of cuts all over my body than ever have skin surgery again.

I immediately thought back to my mom, and I have even more respect for her.

My mom and I have had our ups and downs, but I'm so thankful to her for teaching me to be tough. It's because of her integrity that I'm able to tackle things head on and get through them. I didn't inherit poor genetics from my mom that made me overweight. I inherited a willpower that is as tough as nails.

I want to encourage you to be tough. Know that no matter what obstacle you face, you can get through it.

I LIKE TO SAY TO MYSELF

You're tough.

Chapter 13

#1 Fan

Things eventually started to settle down. We survived in this new kind of normal. I poured myself into the thing I loved most: sports. I loved playing football in high school, but I also loved cheering for the other sports teams at my school as well—especially the basketball team.

Personal determination and skill are critical for an athlete, but I think that sometimes the sideline can be just as important. Having a big cheering squad can boost your confidence as a player. You can use the fans' positive energy as fuel. Big crowds, with lots of encouragement, can really change the outcome of a game.

Because I loved to watch sports and wanted to help the basketball team, I started something called the 6th Man Club. The idea is that a basketball team has five players on the court, and I could be the sixth player on the sideline, screaming and cheering my heart out. After all, the sixth man is essential to the team's success, right?

Well, the 6th Man Club grew from one man, to dozens, and then hundreds. I got all of my friends to stand with me at the games and root for our team. I made sure it was a

52

complete school effort. I would call and text to get everyone there. We had patented cheers. Heck, we were even on the news.

One of my favorite chants was a simple one. We started out slow and quiet, "da da defense... da da defense..." Then we would build, "da da defense... da da defense." Louder still, "DA DA DEFENSE!!! DA DA DEFENSE!!!" until we were screaming and jumping to the rhythm. At this point, I was getting close to 300 pounds, but I still jumped and cheered with everyone else. It was loud, and it was a "look-out-for-us" to the offense. That little chant will always be close to my heart. I can still feel it and hear it ringing in my ears.

The 6th Man Club grew and continued every year I was in school and beyond. Today, they give each incoming freshman a shirt that says: The 6th Man Club.

And here's my point in all of this: Sometimes you've got to be your own sixth man. You've got to cheer for yourself. It's good to find a support system, and I'll talk more about that in a bit. But there will be times when you're on the court of life, and you've got to be able to look on the sidelines and see that number one fan clapping and amping you up!

There will be many moments when you're feeling like you're losing the game. You missed a workout, you went a little crazy on cheat day, you thought negative thoughts. That's when that roar from your own sixth man must be heard (DA DA DEFENSE!). It's the fan on the inside who believes in you. It's the roar that makes you feel like a lion!

I feel like a lion most days now, but that wasn't always the case. I still struggle with old demons. I'll be cruising through the game of life, playing well. But then when things get quiet, and I'm alone with my thoughts, I remember my dad closing that bedroom door. The memories become so vivid that

I can smell him. The flashbacks take over, and pretty soon I've spiraled and started an emotional losing streak. It's in those moments that I have to start up that chant, "da da defense...." I have to keep slowly cheering for myself until the chant gets so loud that I'm able to go back out on the court, give it my all, and win the game.

You've heard the cheers from your sixth man before. I know you have. You probably heard him when you were at a super low point, and you heard that small voice in your head say, "Keep going." That's your sixth man. That's you cheering for yourself! Listen to that man, he knows a lot. And just like a true fan, all he wants for you in your life is to win.

Develop that sixth man (or woman) within yourself so that when you're going through a rough patch, when you have two seconds left on the clock and you're down by two, you can look over at that sixth man, who has so much faith and hope in his eyes, and you can sink a three-pointer.

I LIKE TO SAY TO MYSELF

Cheer for yourself... da da defense!

Chapter 14

You Do You, Boo Boo

*If one advances confidently in the direction of
his dreams, and endeavors to live the life he has
imagined, he will meet with a success unexpected
in common hours.*

— Henry David Thoreau

We all have irrational fears. For me, it's snakes. I can't stand them. I would be happiest if I never saw one again. Even talking about them makes me feel all... (physical shudder with a yuckblah sound).

Fear of snakes is a very common one. Many people are afraid of them. But there is one thing that people are afraid of more than snakes. We all know the study, conducted years ago, that found what it was. The thing that scares people more than dying. Yep, you already guessed it: public speaking. It might terrify you just thinking about it.

While I'm with the masses about thinking snakes are the worst, I'm exactly opposite about public speaking. I actually think it's one of my callings in life. Getting up in front of a large crowd and sharing is all I want to do.

Before the show, before any weight loss, before I told a single soul about my father's abuse, deep down, I was always destined to be a speaker. I think it's because I have always wanted to help people.

There aren't very many speaking opportunities for a high school kid in Provo, Utah. But during my senior year, something truly incredible happened. At graduation it's usually the valedictorian who addresses the crowd, and the class president will say a few words. That's just how it goes. My school wanted to switch things up and allow another student to speak as well. At this point in my life, even though others saw it within me, I didn't know public speaking was my thing. I just thought, "Hey, sure. That sounds fun." There was an audition process, and I pretty much thought it would probably go to someone who was super smart, or super athletic, or just super at something. I wanted to share and inspire my friends and stuff, but I never thought I would actually get to.

I wasn't a 4.0 student. I was probably the furthest from a 4.0 that you could be and still graduate. I remember trying to calculate how many PE classes I could add to help boost my GPA. School has always been a struggle for me, but speaking has always come easy. After they told me I would be standing up in front of everyone at graduation, I began working on my speech. I had a counselor helping me. It was so much fun. I was working toward something and that alone brought me a ton of fulfillment.

It was important to me to have it as memorized as possible. I'm glad I put in the work to do that because on the day of graduation, I was more nervous than I thought I would be. Just because you have a passion doesn't mean you won't have any struggles. I had butterflies. It was nerve-wracking. My hands were cold. I got up on stage—all the lights were on me, blacking out the audience. I took a deep breath, and all of a sudden everything just felt right. It was like something clicked that day. I felt like a normal person up there.

To this day, my coaches, friends, and family remember that speech. I hate talking about it like that because I don't want to sound full of myself or conceited. The whole reason I'm telling you this story is because there is an important truth within it: You must find what you're passionate about and pursue it.

Many people go through life never knowing what their passion is. Forget that. That's not any kind of life worth living. We are all connected by being human, yet there is something special, unique, and different within each one of us. Those differences are what make the world so incredible. There's only one you. You might have something in common with someone else, but remember, there is no one else exactly like you. Embrace that! I believe each of us is born with a calling, a passion, within our heart and a set of tools we can use to pursue that passion. Many people go through life never figuring out what their passion is. They settle for a life that is "safe." It's easier to be average than to be extraordinary. But there's a spark inside every single one of us that gives us the potential to shine bright. When we aren't chasing after something that's bigger than ourselves, it leads to a life that is lacking something.

I know this because it's what happened in my own life. After high school, I started working at a gas station. It helped pay the bills... kind of... more like it made it so we weren't homeless. Was it something I dreamed of doing? No. Was it challenging and rewarding? No. The one thing I liked about that job was that I got to talk to people. That's no surprise! I like talking to people because I care about people. But I couldn't put the dots together back then. I just felt "whatever" about it. That's how life goes. It's so blatantly obvious now that I was meant to develop that love for others and help more than just the regulars at a gas station.

It's very important to take time to figure out who you are and what you feel passionate about. That's the way to live a life of integrity. Even if you never succeed by the world's standards, the pursuit of that dream will bring you life. Quiet your mind, sit in a comfortable spot, or maybe go for a run—whatever you have to do to tune out all the other voices in your head. Get to a mental place where not one distracting thought can get in. Then just wait and listen for the whisper in your heart. What is that little voice saying? Though it may be the quietest, that little heart whisper is the most important voice in your entire life. It's the voice of integrity. Find your calling and run after it.

You are so incredible. There is no one like you! Really work hard to accept those two things. When you live with those positive thoughts, you will start acting differently. You will carry yourself differently. When you feel comfortable and confident in who you are, other people feel it and are inspired by it. How cool is it to see someone who is super into something and have them talk to you about it? Their face lights up. They smile a lot. They may begin talking at a faster pace. It's awesome. You can be like that too.

It's important to dream! Never, ever feel like your dream is stupid. The fact is, most dreams are impractical. They are risky. Does that mean we shouldn't go after them? No! We must! It's not just important to our own well-being, or our integrity, but to the entire world. I'm not trying to be dramatic. I mean that. When we find what we are passionate about and pursue it, I believe we are fulfilling our life's purpose. It's how we can give back to the world. That is what life is all about: giving back.

I LIKE TO SAY TO MYSELF

Find what you love and run toward it.
Be you!

Chapter 15

A Dog's Superpower

After my dad went to prison, our finances took a huge hit. We didn't know what we were going to do. My mom was still working nights, but without my dad's income, we weren't even scraping by, we were just falling behind. I don't really know if it came about because we needed money, or some other reason, but we started breeding dogs. Little, white Maltese dogs. We turned our backyard into the perfect place to breed them. We had a bunch of kennels, a dog run... the works. At any given time, we probably had about fifteen dogs, not including the puppies.

The process was fun, but it was a ton of work. You couldn't leave home for long periods of time. But as hard as it was, it only solidified my love and respect for dogs. Dogs are amazing!

We always had the breeding dogs, but I've also had my own personal dog my whole life. Dogs are the best companions anyone could ever ask for. They are super therapeutic. It doesn't matter what kind of day you're having, they will be happy to see you. They cuddle up next to you. When you walk in the room, it's as if they haven't seen you for years.

Every day is the best day for them. They become a member of your family. They become so special in your heart. It's just amazing what dogs can do. Their love is the definition of unconditional. I have a dog named Zoey now. She's a little rescue and I love her to death. Having dogs be such a big part of my life got me thinking about an awesome characteristic they have: Dogs live in the present.

Something I've struggled with, and continue to struggle with today, is living in the now. Like right now, moment to moment. I worked hard to not dwell in the past. Honestly, through a lot of counseling and hard work, I don't think much about my dad and what happened. I've never wanted to be the victim. But I *do* tend to focus on the future. More specifically, I worry about the future. I literally waste the present day by thinking endlessly about scenarios that usually don't happen. I get so anxious, wondering how the rest of my life will go. And honestly, it's a stupid way to spend my time.

But dogs aren't like that at all. I'll put Zoey in her kennel when I leave, and she will be sad in that moment. But as soon as I get home, she's just excited to see me. She doesn't hold a grudge because I had to leave. No, she soaks up the time we have together in the new moment, in the now. Does Zoey worry about when she will get fed next or if her bed will still be there at night? Absolutely not.

What if humans could act like that? I have to remind myself to just live joyfully in the present. When you think about the past and let it drag you down, or you focus all your energy on the future and it causes you stress, it's a fast track to losing integrity. I have to remember who I am and choose to look at the here and now as an amazing gift. By being like Zoey, and focusing on the present, I'm building my integrity. Every time I banish worries I've made up in my head about the future, or the negative emotions from my past, I am growing as a person. It's not easy living in the now. But I suggest that you try to emulate the unconditionally loving animal that has the superpower of living in the now. Be a dog!

I LIKE TO SAY TO MYSELF

You old dog, you!

Chapter 16

Don't Hide Behind a Mask

My dad was a popular guy. He always had been. He and my mom met doing community theater. He loved that stuff—all the acting and the costumes. My mom did too. She is a really good seamstress, and he was really good at doing costume makeup. They bonded over that.

Having a mom who can sew and a dad who can do awesome makeup meant that I always had the best costumes for Halloween. I challenge you to find another kid in our town who had as realistic costumes as I did. I was Beetlejuice, Leonardo, and the Hulk, just to name a few.

When I was in junior high, I went to school as a werewolf for Halloween. I was walking down the hall when a teacher came up to me and told me about the "no mask" policy for Halloween. He told me I had to take off my mask because rules were rules. I understood the rule. The thing was, I wasn't wearing a mask. My dad had done my makeup, and it looked so good that the teacher thought it was a mask. It wasn't just the face makeup; my dad did my werewolf hair too. He started with a bald cap, blending it perfectly, and then he added the crazy hair.

On that day, everyone thought I was wearing a mask, but I wasn't. In real life, it was the opposite. For years I wore a mask and no one knew.

By not telling anyone that my dad had molested me, too, I had to go out every day and be someone I wasn't. I didn't think like that at the time. I wasn't like, "Oh, time to go out and fool everyone." But when I look back, I can see that's exactly what I was doing. I was hiding. I wasn't able to be truthful, and underneath my exterior, I was dying inside because I wasn't living an authentic life of integrity.

But here is the thing: I actually believed I was fooling people. I'll let you in on a little secret: The people who are close to you know when you're dying inside. The only thing that you can keep from them is the reason why. It's very hard to hide the state of your spirit.

We all have a tendency to act a certain way in public. But I would encourage you to remove any masks you may wear and live authentically. Don't hide from who you are, or from what has happened to you. It doesn't solve anything. It actually makes things worse. Don't be afraid to show the real you. Those who really care about you will stand by you.

I LIKE TO SAY TO MYSELF

No need to hide behind a mask.
You're one good-looking, sound-thinking,
life-changing dude just the way you are.

Chapter 17

Mission Unaccomplished

Growing up in the Church of Jesus Christ of Latter-day Saints (LDS), like any other religion, comes with the many traditions attached to it. One, if not the biggest, is going on a mission. It's a rite of passage from boyhood to manhood (girls go too, but not as many). But more importantly, it's specifically about leading more people to Jesus Christ. Not only does it help the person you're teaching, but since you're going to serve the Lord and make sacrifices, you and your family will be blessed. After high school graduation, for the majority of LDS boys, the next step is going on a mission. Because we lived in the predominately Mormon state of Utah, almost every guy I knew was going on a mission. It's just what you did. So, like the good boy I was always striving to be, after high school, I went on a mission too.

For the first part of your mission, you go to the Missionary Training Center (MTC). The MTC is intense. You're in a group with about twelve other guys. You get up at 6:30 a.m., shower, eat breakfast, go to class, break for lunch, go back to class, break for dinner, go to more class, and then go to bed. Then you wake up and do it all again the next day and the next, for at least two weeks, until you leave for your assigned mission.

The very first day I got there, I felt uncomfortable. School was never my strong suit, so being in a classroom ten hours a day was a challenge. I didn't like the showers. We all had to shower together and it made me feel awkward and embarrassed. Having people see how heavy I was getting was starting to bother me. But there was a deeper reason I was having such a hard time. Back then I didn't know what it was. I just knew I wasn't going to be able to do this. I felt awful. When I look back at it now, I know it's because I was carrying around all this crap from my dad. But at that point in my life, I still hadn't told anyone that he had touched me. In fact, I had adamantly denied it.

On a Friday, three days into my training, I decided to tell them I was leaving. They took me to a special office, and I talked to the president of our group. I told him I wasn't going to be able to make it. He kindly assured me that every missionary goes through these moments and that I was only feeling homesick. "It's normal to feel this way," he said, "It's just the first three days. Once you go through the weekend, you'll be fine." I left his office and tried to convince myself that he was right. I'm never one to quit, so I decided I could do it.

But by the end of the next day, no amount of self-talk was going to keep me there. I couldn't do it. I just felt unsettled. Uneasy. I decided not to go through with it.

The second time I went to the office to tell them I couldn't do it, they had brought in a church leader who was higher up... and my mom. She was LIVID. I think I may have seen actual smoke rising from the top of her head. She demanded to know why I wasn't going on my mission. Man, she was fuming that day.

The higher-up guy was a little calmer. "Why are you going home?" he asked. I couldn't even answer that question myself, let alone give an answer to someone else. Underneath his calm exterior, I knew he was angry with me. He went on, "You know, people who don't finish their LDS missions usually end up where your dad is." My mom looked at me and was nodding her head in agreement. "I don't know. I'm sorry. I just can't do it," was all I could get out. What they were implying scared me.

On our way to the car, I was no longer safe within the confines of a church building, and my mom laid into me. She was screaming and yelling. She continued to criticize me for not completing my mission—ranting on and on, the whole way home.

Things with my mom didn't get better. While I didn't like her approach, I could see where she was coming from. Her whole life was the LDS church. She didn't know anything different. It really divided my mom and me, big time. She told me I was a let-down. I knew I was letting her down, but what I couldn't explain to her was that I was letting myself down more. No one could see that I was dying inside.

Maybe it was because of routine, or familiarity, or to make up for leaving my mission, but I went to church on Sunday. The church always preached about loving one another and building each other up. I thought I could find comfort in my church community. I was wrong.

Some members that I had known my whole life were turning on me. Some were subtle, just giving me judgmental looks, but others showed brazen disappointment. One old-school guy said to me, "I told my son not to come home unless it was in a body bag." Thankfully, not many people treated me like this.

I decided to get some guidance from our bishop. He was one of the people who showed kindness and understanding toward me. He told me it was okay and that he supported me. That's the way people are supposed to be. I don't blame the religion for the negative onslaught I received; I blame some of the people in it. As in any religion, the religion itself isn't the problem, the flawed people are. And let's be honest: We're all flawed in one way or another, and that's why we go to church—to become better.

I went home and my mom was still very critical. I didn't want to be around all that negativity, so I tried to stay with some good friends. Surely they would understand and just joke around like always. But just like some of the other supporters in my life, they began to bail on me. Some guys even said to me, "Until you go back on your mission, we're not going to hang out with you." I was bouncing around from couch to couch like a nomad. I felt like a leper.

I didn't know what to do. I had lost everything and everyone... except one. There was still one person left who I knew would understand where I was coming from. The one person who I thought truly loved me: my dad.

In the state prison, there were three visiting days: Tuesday, Saturday, and Sunday. I made up my mind to go there on a Saturday. Jail is not a place you want to visit. Visiting hours were from 8:00–10:00 a.m., but you had to get there at least an hour early to go through all of the security and get checked in. You went through gate after gate, offering your ID every time. Then you'd go through the metal detector. They would run your name and make sure everything was clear. All the while, every employee just looked like they didn't want to be there and eyed you like "Why are you here?" All the visitors would line up against a wall and wait to go through all the gates. The whole process makes you feel like an inmate. Finally, you could go sit and wait in the visiting room. I was at a giant, round table that probably would seat six to eight people.

Other people were meeting an inmate, too, but you never really paid attention to them because you were always so focused on the person you were there to see. I was especially focused on that day.

They brought out all the inmates in a single-file line. I saw my dad in his white jumpsuit with a look of surprise on his face. He didn't expect to see me because, as far as he knew, I was still at the MTC. He sat down, and I told him everything. I poured my heart out to the one person I felt safest around. I explained how the stress got to me and I had to leave early. I confessed that I didn't think it was my time, but I was going to try and get back out on my mission soon. I questioned aloud why I left and how I didn't understand it. Finally, I finished by saying, "Dad, I was thinking you would understand and know what to do." Then I took a breath and waited for my dad to respond. I already felt a bit better.

My dad's reply hit me like a ton of bricks, knocking all the air from my lungs again. He was cold as ice, and his words were piercing: "Well, son, I just think the family is not going to receive the blessings we deserve. Now it's your fault I'm in here. Because you did this, I'm not ever going to get out of here. I was counting on those blessings."

I have never felt so weak. I just sat there. It was all that negative talk—all that judgment I had felt growing up. It brought back all those feelings that were hiding just under the surface—feelings of inadequacy. All I wanted was to be the best son I could be. But here it was again that I was a failure. I felt awful. My dad got in my head. So many kids have gone on their missions, and I'm not going like I'm supposed to.

I left the prison. Because I lost my last and strongest supporter, I began questioning the worth of my life. It felt like there was no reason for me to be around. If I was such a disappointment and failure to everyone, wouldn't it be better for everyone if I wasn't around?

Not only that, but my dad turned my faith. He twisted it and distorted it, just like he does with everything else. He made me feel like God was mad at me.

For the next couple of days, all I could think about was how alone I felt—no friends, no family, no church, no God. Then I remembered my cousin.

About two years before this point, he killed himself. He hanged himself. I thought, "Okay, that's what I could do." My cousin was free from his pain. I could be too. When you're in such a dark place, you lose all rational thought. You see the whole world through a muted lens. All color has drained from your view. Food loses its flavor. You drift through your day like a zombie. I wasn't fully present. If I had been thinking clearly, maybe I would've remembered that in my cousin's suicide note he alluded to my dad sexually molesting him as well. It never occurred to me that my father's actions might have been the cause of his suicide. Or that if I killed myself, then that would be another win for the enemy. Two souls would've been gone forever because of my dad. But I wasn't thinking clearly. I didn't realize that my cousin and I were not suffering because of something we had done, but because of something that was done to us.

I wish I could go back in time and talk to my cousin before he took his own life. I wish I could've shown him that life gets better, and that through a lot of hard work and love, you can overcome what happened to you. I would give anything to tell him it wasn't his fault.

No one got to me in time either. Because things were still bad with my mom, and I wasn't staying at the house, I snuck home a couple of nights after seeing my dad and crept down to the basement. The steps were familiar. They were the steps I walked down at night with my dad for over six years. I drank a big old bottle of booze. The biggest one I could find. We had a hammock hook-up downstairs, so I got a belt and tied it to the hook. I stood on a chair and put the belt around my neck. Then I jumped. I'm still here to tell the story, I'm still alive, because of one thing: my weight. I was so heavy that the belt broke. In this rare instance, being overweight actually saved my life.

I sat on the floor and began to cry.

I LIKE TO SAY TO MYSELF

No matter how hopeless it feels, it gets better.

Chapter 18

Coach Olsen

"You dumbass! Don't you know that you've got friends and people that you can rely on? This isn't the answer! What were you thinking?!" Coach Olsen admits that he wasn't very nice to Bruce when he went to visit him in the hospital the night of Bruce's suicide attempt. "I felt like, at that time, he needed a swift kick in the butt to let him know that there were people that loved him. This is not the way to do things." As a man who cared about Bruce like a father to a son, Donny Olsen was upset.

It was in the hospital, when he was still very intoxicated, that Bruce couldn't hold it in any longer and admitted to everyone what his father had done to him. In a moment, everything clicked for Olsen: all of Bruce's behavior, his weight gain, leaving his mission, all of it made sense. Olsen was beyond angry with Danny Pitcher, hardly able to express his rage. "When I found out that this was what happened to Bruce... if his dad were in the room, I would've kicked... I would've just gone off. Nobody deserves that."

Donny Olsen is still a high school football coach, and he has a successful career in the mortgage industry. His house has all the grandness that you would expect from a guy who knows real estate, but with an incredibly warm and homey feel. You want to just sit on his couch and never leave. Donny says he owes it to his wife and jokes that he's responsible for the weeds. He's doing a good job because his perfectly manicured lawn doesn't have a weed in sight. Looking at his cozy home and his loving family, you can't help but compare it to Bruce's childhood home, with all its clutter and coldness. It's not hard to put together why Bruce would go to the Olsen house to watch the game on a Saturday and stay all day.

It was sophomore year, the year his father went to prison, that Bruce met Coach Olsen, who was head coach. At first, Olsen only saw the happy-go-lucky Bruce that everyone instantly connected with. "But then some things started happening through the year. Kids that age, boys that age, can be cruel. Back then, Bruce had a real good group of friends, but then there were some that weren't such good guys, that really didn't know Bruce." Olsen explained that some of the other players would "torment Bruce." But being a caring and seasoned coach, Olsen put a stop to it almost immediately. He brought the players together and threatened to dismantle the team. His stern approach worked. "After that everyone came together. That's when everyone came to his rescue."

Throughout Bruce's high school years, Coach Olsen, along with everyone else, noticed how much Bruce loved life. On the outside, Bruce seemed to be the life of the party, but on the inside, he was harboring some serious demons. At home, Bruce struggled, but he tried to hide it from Olsen and the other coaches. "Bruce would have bad days... He wouldn't say what was bothering him, but you could just tell he wasn't himself." Olsen describes how he and the other coaches chose to be proactive and help Bruce even when he didn't ask. Olsen knew Bruce's home life wasn't always great. The coach could also recognize the situation: "His mom, bless her heart—how do you react to that type of news? She didn't take it very well and she took it out on Bruce. That wasn't right. There were times when we had to pull Bruce out of his house. It wasn't a good environment." Olsen helped arrange places for Bruce to stay when things would get a bit too heated with his mom.

Just like everyone else, the more Olsen got to know Bruce, the more he suspected that maybe he had been abused by his father as well. But as open and honest as Bruce was, he was never able to talk about the one thing that was plaguing him. "That's where all the problems started," Olsen explains. "When you don't start talking about things, then you can't really address the issues." The coach was spot-on in his assessment, but adds humbly, "Of course, I'm no psychologist."

But given all of that, the ever-joyful Bruce almost never let his personal life interfere with his social life at school. Olsen knows that Bruce was selected to speak at graduation because he was such a beloved and active student. Bruce's energy levels never seemed to be depleted. His genuine love and enthusiasm were always readily available to anyone.

After high school, Coach Olsen credits Coach Wong for getting Bruce involved in coaching almost immediately. When Wong appointed him to the position, Olsen could see why it was such a good fit. "Bruce is knowledgeable. He knows what he's talking about when it comes to football. He really does... Bruce knows what he's doing when it comes to coaching. The kids love him. The kids just warm up to him because he's so enthusiastic. You can tell he loves what he's doing."

It seemed like everything was turning around for Bruce after high school. However, his dad's abuse still haunted him, and the secret ate at him. Bruce had always been a bigger kid, which was helpful when he played linebacker, but after high school he really began to pack on the pounds. Olsen jokes at first, saying they would get wings and all kinds of food. But he gets more serious when he says, "We were concerned." Olsen wasn't alone in trying to help Bruce shed some pounds, but without knowing the real cause of this weight gain, their advice fell on deaf ears. "The way Bruce's life was going, he was still the happy-go-lucky guy. He was still coaching and still doing those fun things that he wanted to do, but his life was going to be short. He was going in a direction that wasn't going to last."

However, the weight wasn't the biggest concern. Olsen never knew quite how bad things were for Bruce emotionally until he got the call that Bruce was in the hospital. When he got there he was so disappointed that Bruce didn't call him or any of his other friends, saying, "Why didn't you come see me? Why didn't we talk it out? Instead of taking such a big step?" All he wanted was to be there for Bruce.

Chapter 19

Speak

I don't know if it was because of the alcohol, being in the hospital, or having a complete breakdown. But one good thing that came out of my suicide attempt was that it caused me to finally say what I had been through with my dad.

My dad went to prison when I was fourteen years old. I was twenty before I told anyone I had been abused. For six years I was just holding it in. When you don't talk about traumatic experiences that are bothering you, a strange thing happens. The longer you don't say anything, the more you think you're becoming okay with whatever you're not talking about. But it's actually the exact opposite. The unspoken things will begin to live and grow inside you. Every day you have to push more and more things down. You can try to ignore them. But deep down, where all the grit and grime is, you know you're not overcoming them, you're just avoiding them.

In the beginning, I was keeping the secret for my dad. I was scared he would go to prison. I didn't want to lose him. He had told me to keep the secret, and I did what he said. But after he was locked up—while he still influenced me, big time—I began not talking because I was afraid of what people might think. Child abuse messes with your head. You don't know where the truth is. People tell you how bad and how shameful the abuse is. They are scolding the accuser, but it's hard not to feel dirty and guilty yourself for what happened. It's hard to reconcile that, even though you participated, it was done to you. It's taken me a long time to learn that I didn't actually make the choice to have my dad molest me. My dad wanted me to think that. He wanted me to think it was consensual. But I was a vulnerable and impressionable child. I didn't make that choice at all. When I was younger, I couldn't understand that. I didn't want to tell people because I was worried they would judge me. Simple as that.

Finally talking about what happened to me was the biggest weight off of my shoulders. I can't describe it. Nothing was solved. There weren't even any scars yet, just open wounds. But with the help of professionals and those who cared about me, I could begin to tackle the situation head-on. I was on the road to integrity.

After my suicide attempt, I spent two weeks in the psychiatric wing of the hospital. It was the perfect place for me to be. The thing that stands out the most to me was how understanding everyone was. All my fears were a lie. They were fears my dad instilled in me. If you're going through a tough time, don't be afraid to ask for help. I received so much help in those two weeks.

It's good for you to speak about your demons because your silence is keeping you from getting fit and healthy. Until you're ready to talk about your issues, you won't be able to lose weight and keep it off.

But speaking doesn't just help you, it helps those around you. Even though I was like this Jolly Green Giant, everyone knew something was up with me. They were almost helpless to help me because they had no idea what the heck was going on. That's completely unfair.

While the importance of talking things through applies to the serious issues, it also applies to your daily grind. Years later, when I was on *Extreme Weight Loss*, I was having a hard day. My attitude was not good. That's when Heidi Powell, co-host of the show and the sweetest lady I know, stepped in and said, with some tough love, "You see what you're doing now? Look at your mood right now. Look at everyone's mood right now. This is our life and your spirit. When you're down, it affects the entire group." That was a wake-up call to me. It brought me back to what I learned the two weeks I was in the hospital. I opened up to Heidi about what was bothering me, we talked it out, and then I was able to go back and crush it! I knew that because of what I went through, and what I learned, I couldn't be like that. God gave me my life to inspire people, and I wasn't going to waste it by storing up negative feelings again.

You can't waste your life by being silent either. Speaking out won't be the ultimate fix, but it is the first step toward recovery and life-long healing.

I LIKE TO SAY TO MYSELF

Tell people what you're going through.

Chapter 20

Skyler

Skyler and Bruce met on the field at a pick-up flag football game. They were on opposite teams and Bruce tried to fight Skyler. They both laugh thinking about it now. "Bruce was always just passionate about winning," Skyler says with a little smile.

They had barely graduated from high school when they met each other. Realizing they are now in their thirties, Skyler is stunned and can't figure out where the time has gone. Over the past decade, Skyler has been there for Bruce like a brother. His temperament is the polar opposite of Bruce's. Bruce can rile up a crowd, but Skyler is calm and content. He has a surfer vibe, even though he was born and raised in Utah. He wears his sandals as often as he can.

Bruce said their friendship grew really strong, really quickly. When asked what good qualities Bruce has, Skyler is quick to describe his best friend: "Bruce is just a fun-loving guy. Everybody knows him. Everybody loves him. He's passionate about whatever he's doing in the moment. He cares about everybody. He cares about how they feel. He's always open to opinions." Skyler admits that many people feel like they are Bruce's best friend, because that's just how Bruce makes you feel when you're around him.

And Skyler has been through it all with Bruce. He has seen Bruce's highest highs and lowest lows. But one thing Skyler emphasizes is how Bruce is larger than life. "He's fun to be around. He's always up for anything. Even when he was big, he was up for doing things that probably big guys shouldn't have been doing." Bruce was a party anywhere he went.

Skyler tells a story about when the Utah Jazz had a contest to find the biggest Jazz fan. All you had to do was send in a picture. "So we went over to my house... This was back when Bruce was kinda getting big... and we got him all dressed up." Bruce had a jersey, a cape, a homemade helmet—the works. "We even had my dog dressed up in a little Jazz getup." That picture captured the genuine love that Bruce had for the Jazz, and he won four tickets. They weren't just any tickets, though, "they were $1,000 seats in the Alexis box." The prized seats came with a fancy dinner, almost on the floor of the court. Bruce, Skyler, and Skyler's two brothers had a blast. Typical Bruce went over the top in his cheering and jeering. "The whole time we were right behind the Bulls announcers. We were yelling and cheering the whole time. I was getting text messages from people watching and they were telling us that the announcers were telling the four people behind them to shut up because they couldn't hear. They couldn't even hear the announcers commentating on the game. We went back and looked on ESPN... we were the topic of many discussions."

Bruce loved hanging out at Skyler's house. Skyler's family had all the love and welcoming acceptance that Bruce craved, but never received, from his own father. Bruce always seemed to have trouble with cars. Skyler recounts when he was driving with Bruce and they got pulled over on the free-way. Bruce's car didn't have proper registration, so the officer took the vehicle right then and there, leaving the friends to walk home. "I vowed to never drive with Bruce again," Skyler laughs.

That was alright because Skyler had a little moped. "I remember when I used to go down in Provo and take my scooter, my moped, to pick him up. It was like *Dumb and Dumber*. We topped out at 20–25 mph, and we were on like a 50 mph road and everyone was honking at us. We were just going to my house. I went and picked him up and brought him back." Skyler explains that the trip, which should take about twenty minutes, took nearly forty-five minutes.

Skyler initially became close with Bruce because he felt compassion for a person that had been through so much. "I continued to help him because he was a good friend. He's one of those guys where you really feel for his situation. I come from a family where my parents are married. My dad has a good job. I haven't had to want. If I needed things, those things were available. Whereas you see someone like Bruce, where he doesn't have a car. He got the short end of the stick, so you root for him and try and help him. You feel like you want to help him out and give him opportunities." But Skyler stayed close with Bruce because of his fun-loving, caring personality. "The good stuff outweighed the negative times you had with him." And now, Skyler experiences mostly good times with Bruce. There is a deep love between the two men. When asked what Skyler likes most about Bruce, he explains, "I would just say he's got a great personality. He's always in a great mood."

Chapter 21

Nick

"Honestly, to be friends with Bruce at that time was a burden." That's what Bruce's friend Nick had to say when he joined in the conversation with Skyler. Nick met Bruce around the same time as Skyler. While Skyler recognized Bruce's enthusiasm for life, he could also attest to Nick's sentiments. It was clear to both friends that Bruce was struggling, even with his outgoing personality.

It wasn't that long after they met Bruce that it finally came out that his father had molested him as well. Bruce's mom was struggling too and not treating Bruce very well. Nick was the friend Bruce stayed with after his failed attempt to go on his mission. Nick talks about that time: "[Bruce] was at a low point in his life. He would literally lie in bed all day. He didn't have a job. Didn't have anything going for him." Seeing his friend like this wasn't easy for Nick. "It was hard for me to watch. It was hard to see my friend just wasting away in my bedroom."

When Bruce was out and about, hanging out with his friends, things were much better. "Don't get me wrong, I love the kid to death, and I would do anything for him, but it was a task to take care of Bruce," Nick says. He describes the fights Bruce would start and the fits of rage Bruce would have. One time, Bruce punched a sign and it was so loud that the cops showed up because a neighbor thought that a gun had been fired. Another time, the friends were standing under a streetlight and some guys they didn't know told them to leave. Bruce started yelling and throwing rocks at them.

Sometimes the fights were over more important things. Nick tells a story about a time they were all at a community pool. A guy was dunking his girlfriend under water. He was holding her down too long, and when she would surface, she was crying and screaming for him to stop. "She was terrified. Bruce, before anybody, just rushed over there and destroyed this kid. Because he had that nature, that protective nature." Nick also notes that Bruce's weight, around 350 pounds, was a huge advantage. Still, Nick says, "I don't want to sound like all we did was fight."

Bruce also had crippling insecurities. While it may have taken Bruce a while to understand where that stemmed from, Nick and Skyler knew it was because he was always searching for his father's approval. Nick explains that Bruce was going through the darkest time of his life, but he would swing from the highest highs to the lowest lows, something Nick felt was manic-depressive behavior. When Bruce would get "really low," Nick and his friends said, "That's when you had to reassure him emotionally and say, 'No, you're a good guy. We love you. We want you to be around us. We want you to be here. You're one of our best friends.' I can't tell you how many conversations I had with him like that."

Before Bruce got on *Extreme Weight Loss* things didn't really get much better. He continued to get in fights and needed to be reassured all the time. However, Nick makes sure to bring up that if you're a friend of Bruce, he'll be there for you no matter what. "He might need to be picked up to get there, but he'll be there." The thing Nick likes the most about Bruce that hasn't ever changed is his love for people: "He never makes people feel bad. I know I've made him feel bad. But I don't think one time he's ever made me feel bad about myself. He doesn't put people down. He doesn't put anyone down. And in our friend group, that's what we do. Somehow, he's survived it all, but never jumped in with it."

What's also clear to Nick, and those around Bruce, is how his life has turned around since the show. "Something that I really love now is that I call him for advice. That's one of my favorite things in the world. Now I can call Bruce, who used to be 400 pounds, and get advice about my diet and working out. He's probably the last person on earth that I thought I would call about that stuff." Another positive thing to come for Bruce? "He doesn't have his temper like he used to. That changed after the show." Those fits of anger, rooted in his subconscious rage toward his father, don't plague Bruce anymore. And Bruce got his confidence back because of the show. "Not only does he look different, like, he is literally a different person. He's happier. The show truly changed his life."

Chapter 22

No Idea

I t would be a long time before I became the new man I am today. The man who Nick talks about as being a different person. After high school, I was struggling. I missed football. Because of my insane passion for and knowledge of the game, my former high school coaches thought it seemed like a perfect fit for me to help coach the team. I was stoked. It was hard being away from it. Plus, I was hanging around my coaches all the time anyway.

It was not until I decided to write this book that I found out something about my coaches and the city that I never knew before. Coach Wong explained that when some members of the community found out I would be assistant coaching, they were not happy. The news about my dad being a child molester had been public knowledge for a long time, and my own admission of being abused by my dad was slowly circulating as well. Parents felt super uncomfortable that I would be around their young sons. Sadly, I guess it's common for victims to follow in their abuser's footsteps. That sickens me and I can't understand it. But a lot of people in the town were fueled by fear and wanted me fired immediately.

Still completely unbeknownst to me, a town meeting was held to determine whether I would be allowed to coach or not. My coaches really went to bat for me. Coach Wong said, "I basically told the community to stuff it. Bruce was under my watch. I just said, 'Nope, Bruce would never do that.' I wasn't concerned at all because I knew Bruce. If I had any doubts, I wouldn't have let him do it, but I knew he was alright." The people either believed my coaches, or simply caved, because I became an assistant coach.

Hearing this story only recently has had a profound effect on me. While my coaches' belief in me is humbling and makes me feel good, it floors me to think that people felt so strongly. It hurts. I guess I shouldn't be that surprised. I know it's a stigma against me. The prejudice is most noticeable when I'm around kids. As soon as I begin interacting in any way with children, I can feel eyes on me. Normally, I don't pay attention to what other people think, but their judgment is so strong, it's palpable. My dad's sins are still haunting me. I still have to carry his weight.

Chris and Heidi Powell, hosts of *Extreme Weight Loss*, have no problem with me being around their kids. I love those four little kids to death. Many of my friends back home have kids. My friend Skyler says I'm great with his two boys.

But all of that positive feedback feels like a drop in the bucket compared to all the strangers. I'm discouraged that others might think I would harm a child in any way. I love kids!

But it brings up a point that you have to understand to be able to move forward: There are always going to be people who think something about you that's a lie. It's because there will always be judgment in the world. One of my friends told me something Aristotle said that makes a lot of sense to me:

"To avoid criticism, say nothing, do nothing, be nothing." We are all going to be criticized unjustly. It won't be fair. I mean, seriously, do I deserve to be judged because of what my father did to me? Absolutely not. But I can't waste my time dwelling on what people think of me. Because even if I try the hardest I can possibly try, and live a life of integrity, some people would *still* think those lies about me. You've just got to let it go.

I've decided to act normally and live a good life, a life full of integrity. That's all I can do. I won't convince them with my words, but my actions will speak for me. I don't want to have to try and work so hard to gain everyone's trust. I know I'm trustworthy. It's up to them if they want to see that or not. It really is their problem, not mine.

I LIKE TO SAY TO MYSELF

Don't think about the haters.
You're awesome!

Chapter 23

Take a Sick Day

I wish I could say that after my first suicide attempt I never tried something so stupid and selfish ever again, but I can't. I had finally admitted what my dad had done, but I still carried the burden of it with me everywhere I went.

Coach Clark said I was a lost sheep. I felt like it. High school was over. I would never go on my mission. My daily high school football practices stopped, so I started gaining a lot of weight. I found a job at the gas station and worked part time as a football coach. I resigned myself to the fact that that was all my life was ever going to be. We all go through seasons in our lives, and that was a dark one for me. I had more good days than bad, but a lot of days the only thing I looked forward to was eating. A bag of Doritos, or a few candy bars, or my personal favorite, Reese's Pieces, would bring me comfort. Thinking my life was going nowhere (which was a total lie), I needed a lot of comfort, which meant I needed a lot of food. I really started packing on the pounds with this coping mechanism. I was nearing 400 pounds. The heavier I got, the worse I felt; the more I ate to comfort myself, the heavier I got... you get the idea. It was a vicious cycle.

Now that I am out of that place, I have the ability to look back with a clear heart and mind and learn from it. Like, one day I was just sitting on my couch and BOOM! I thought of something I had never thought of before. You know what insight I've found? It's okay to take mental sick days. Everything isn't always hunky-dory. We have sick days for our bodies, but why don't we have sick days for our spirit?

Think about what happens when you get physically sick. There are times when, no matter how well I take care of myself, I end up getting a cold or something. I get all the sleep I need. I feed my body well. I work out like the healthiest of Americans. I even wash my hands like I learned in grade school. Yet, somehow, I get the flu, and it knocks me out. There was nothing I could've done differently. So when my nose begins running, or my temperature spikes, and my body is shutting down, I give it the physical rest it needs. I call in a sick day. I take the time I need to recuperate and boost my immune system. Why is it different when I am sick emotionally? Or mentally?

All of us will have rough days. Some inexplicable, some caused by an obvious source, but all of them bring us down one way or another. When you try to make a big change in your life, mental setbacks like this can be seen as weaknesses. It's completely discouraging to be discouraged! However, it's so important to remember to let yourself have a rough moment. Sometimes I just say, "I'm not feeling it today."

After trying to kill myself, I had a lot of days like that. There were so many moments where I wasn't feeling it. But I never gave up entirely. I had to remember that I wasn't failing by taking time to recuperate my spirit. It's just like resting when you have a cold; you will get better. You can't stay in your sick bed for your entire life, but allow healing to occur.

You have a right to be upset sometimes, but don't play the "poor me" card.

Here's another analogy that helped me understand the idea of taking an emotional sick day without falling off the wagon entirely: Pack your bags, but don't leave. As much as the show was a huge blessing to me, there were times when I wanted to quit. I could get pumped and help others, but some weeks I wouldn't lose as much as I wanted or not lose at all, and I couldn't take it. I thought about leaving, but I didn't.

When you embark on something so big, it's easy to feel pressure. Not even from others, but just from yourself. You want to keep your promises and keep your integrity, but on those days when you know you can't, you fall even further because you're disappointed. Don't let an emotional sick day last longer than it needs to because you're upset that you took a day at all. No, take the sick day, and then get back on that horse!

I LIKE TO SAY TO MYSELF

It's okay to take an emotional sick day.

Chapter 24

Bailey

Bailey laughs nervously when she's asked about the first moment she met Bruce. The story is "so Bruce," which means that it includes potty humor. She was eighteen years old and had just moved to Provo to start her freshman year at BYU. Bruce was twenty at the time.

"'I know it's happened to you,'" Bailey hesitantly begins to tell the first thing Bruce said to her. They were at a little party and Bruce had just walked up, "'You've gone number two and wiped, but the toilet paper broke and a little bit of poop got on your finger... so you smelled it! You know you've smelled it!'" Bailey says she knows it was a crude story, but that's how Bruce was sometimes. It was endearing. From that moment on, Bailey instantly liked Bruce. He was hilarious and had an almost childlike, caring nature.

One time, Bailey and Bruce went to the movies. It was a comedy. Bruce was laughing so loud and slapping his knee so hard that Bailey was almost embarrassed by his behavior... but not really. She loved that about him.

However, it wasn't long before Bailey began to see the darker side of the guy who was larger than life. "I learned about his dad early on... We were driving by the prison and Bruce pointed and said, 'My dad's in there.'" Bruce told Bailey the story everyone knew: His dad had molested many little boys. But his darkest secret was still very much hidden... or so Bruce thought. "I knew deep down something had happened to him. I would ask him over and over again. He would deny it every time," said Bailey. But she thought some of Bruce's behavior was giving him away: "He wasn't comfortable giving hugs to me. He had a hard time saying 'I love you' back."

Bailey's relationship with Bruce was complicated. While Bruce may have struggled to say it, an instant connection and deep love ran between them, even though things always stayed platonic. Bruce trusted Bailey, and because they were so close, she was the first person he told about his father molesting him. Bailey said to him, "I know this happened to you," over and over until he finally admitted it. Even though it wasn't a surprise, the truth was painful to hear. To this day, Bailey admits, "When I think about what Bruce went through, it brings tears to my eyes. I can't help but cry. I also get emotional because I was closest to Bruce when he was going through one of the hardest seasons in his life."

Bailey was very much a part of the night Bruce tried to kill himself. After failing at hanging himself, he was falling over drunk, crying and yelling at his dad (who wasn't there, but just a figment of his imagination), saying, "How could you do this to me? I miss you." To Bailey's horror, Bruce went out on the busy road in front of the house, still crying and yelling, talking to his dad. Bailey said he was belligerent, "I didn't know what to do. I was worried he would get hit by a car. I didn't know how to stop him. So I thought, if I push him over, he's not going to be able to get up." That's exactly what she did. Then Bailey called the man who loved Bruce like a son: Coach Clark. He came and called the police, and they took Bruce to the hospital.

After Bruce admitted out loud to everyone what his dad had done to him, Bailey noticed that he was able to talk about it more easily. But the road to recovery would be a long one, and Bailey was set on helping him any way she could. It wasn't an easy thing for an eighteen-year-old freshman to handle. Bailey admits she didn't have the tools, just a great love for someone she considered a brother. Bruce had trouble with counseling at first, so Bailey went with him to sessions. "He didn't want to talk to people because that terrified him." She tried hard to be there for him. However, hurts that deep don't go away overnight. "Even though he went to therapy, things weren't fixed."

Things got so bad her father began to worry about her. "He would say, 'You need to distance yourself. You need to get away from him.'" These seem like harsh words now, but at the time, it was advice based on the reality of the situation.

Everyone who is close to Bruce knows he tried to commit suicide once. But less than a handful know that he tried to take his own life not once, not twice, but many, many times. And nearly every time it was Bailey who found out first.

"We talked practically every day, so I would always get a bad feeling when I didn't hear from him. Many times, I would get in my car, drive to his house, and find him in his room, in the basement, trying to do the unthinkable. It was terrifying." Bailey describes, through tears, one particularly bad attempt: "I found him trying to hang himself again. Blood vessels were broken in his head. He was purple. I knew it was a cry for help, but as a nineteen-year-old, I didn't know what to do." Bailey was so afraid for Bruce.

Bailey saw a hurting person, whose emotional state swung like a pendulum. "When he was okay, he was so okay. But when he was low, he was so low." For many years Bailey was with Bruce through his darkest times. But through everything, she also got to know the funny guy with the crude jokes. The guy she met at the party her freshman year. "Everything he does, he does with full passion. He doesn't do anything halfway." Even though Bruce was fighting his demons, he still managed to be there for Bailey too. He helped her get a job at Costco. He was there to comfort her when her father died suddenly in a car accident. He loved in the ways he knew how.

Today, Bailey is living in Utah, married with two kids. She talks about her friendship with Bruce with wisdom and clarity. They are forever bonded from the years they spent working through his darkest days together.

Chapter 25

Go Lakers!* (*Not)

Something that has helped me my entire life, but especially when I was shedding the extra pounds, has been to keep my word. It's a big part of your integrity. When you do what you say you are going to do, you become more honorable. To have honor makes you a better human being. Keeping my word has helped me in three ways:

1. It causes me to think before I speak. All of the promises spoken out of my mouth will have authenticity. I might take an extra moment to think through what I'm about to say. Giving an idea more thought always makes for a better idea. It helps me cast aside negative statements or foolish thoughts. If I know that I must keep my word no matter what, I'm going to filter what I promise and determine whether I can actually stay true to my word.

2. It will hold me accountable. If I accept this principle, then I will be more likely to stick to the steps toward living with integrity. If I say I'm going to the gym, then I'm going to keep my word and go to the gym. Simple as that! If I say I'm going to cut back on refined sugar,

then I'm going to keep my word and avoid soda. This concept needs to permeate you to your core as well. Those thoughts you have, but don't speak, are words and promises you're making to yourself. So if you make a declaration that you're going to banish bad thoughts from your mind, then stop putting yourself down in your head. No one else may be able to hear you breaking your word, but you will. Hold yourself accountable too.

3. It fosters trust between me and my friends. No one likes a flake. If I prove to my friends that I will do what I say I will do, they will think better of me and will often reciprocate. If you try it, it will help you form closer bonds and have an even better support group. If you have a workout plan or a life plan, and you keep your word and follow it, your friends will feel inspired by it. They will know you're a person of honor and integrity.

Here's a little story about how I went to the utmost extreme to keep my word and keep my integrity. I was twenty-three at the time, working at the gas station, living life, and loving sports. Probably tipping the scales at around 350 pounds. On the radio, they were talking about how the Utah Jazz was going to play the LA Lakers in the second round of the NBA playoffs. Before we can continue, you must understand: I can't decide if I love the Jazz more than I hate the Lakers, or if I hate the Lakers more than I love the Jazz. Let's put it this way, the team I loved most in the entire world was going to play the team that I would rather have eradicated from the earth. So I called up the radio station to tell them the Jazz would destroy the Lakers and obtain victory. I was positive. I told them, "If the Jazz don't win game three in Salt

Lake City, I will get a Lakers tattoo." I swore it on my life. Cross my heart, hope to die.

Well, the short story is the Jazz lost. But I wasn't about to break my promise. I would keep my word and get that Lakers tattoo. But on the day I was going to get inked, something terrible happened. My mom called me to say that she found my dog, Mitsy, dead in the middle of the road. She had been hit by a car. We were breeding dogs, but Mitsy was my dog. I was devastated. I started crying. I told my mom I couldn't go through with the tat. It was just too much. My mom, tough as nails, said, "Bruce, you made a promise to those listeners and to yourself, and you better keep your word!" I couldn't believe it. Then she said, "I'll clean up the mess, and you get that tattoo!" It was the bucket of ice water I needed to jar me back to reality.

Now I have the logo of my least favorite team in the entire world tattooed on my upper thigh. It's kind of big. I suppose I could've made it a little smaller, but that's beside the point. Every morning when I get dressed and see that tattoo, it doesn't remind me of how much I hate the Lakers. It reminds me that I kept my word. And in a weird way, it makes me feel proud of myself.

If I can keep my word and be permanently marked for the rest of my life with something I hate, then you can keep your word too.

I LIKE TO SAY TO MYSELF

Nice tat. Nice job keeping your word.

Chapter 26

Naked Squats

G et yourself pumped up! Ignite the day!

I want to let you in on a little secret. It's simple. It's short. It's not something that needs a huge chapter devoted to it. It's something I do almost every morning. I started doing it long before I lost weight. I made it a part of my morning ritual to ignite the day. I have two words for you: naked squats.

Here's the deal: Weight loss is a mental game, so it's important to get yourself pumped every morning before you start the day and every moment you're feeling down. My alarm goes off and the day begins, baby! I shoot out of bed and take hold of the new dawn by both horns. I go to the bathroom, strip down, and do some naked squats right there in front of my mirror. It gets my blood flowing. It makes me feel alive. And it will make you feel alive too!

I look at myself in the mirror and pump myself up: "You can do this, Bruce!" "You're a fighter, Bruce!" "Seize the day! Have integrity! Be kind! Let's rock this!!!" I talk to myself like I would talk to a team before a big game. I would do this when I was over 400 pounds. Not to be crude, but I would stand in front of that mirror, naked as the day I came into this world, and say, "You're one handsome dude!" "I wonder what the ladies will think today." It worked for me to say things like that. It helped my self-esteem. Because, let's face it, being so overweight, I didn't have very much of it.

It sounds so stupid, but it worked for me. If you wait for your emotional state to change, you may be waiting forever. But if you choose action, the emotions often follow.

I LIKE TO SAY TO MYSELF

Do some naked squats!

Chapter 27

Respect Your Locker Room

I lived at the same address for over two decades. If you drove by, all you would see was an unassuming little white house. It had a single-car carport to the left and six steps, lined with white railing, that led to the front porch on the right. There were only three windows on the front of the house: two vertical ones on either side of the front door and one big one to the left of that. It was my home, and the only home I had ever known. After all the allegations came out and my dad went to prison, we continued to live in that house. We didn't have anywhere else to go and money was tight. I didn't think it bothered me at the time, but looking back, I think it would've been better to get out of there sooner than we did. To be walking around and living among so many bad memories wasn't healthy or helpful in moving forward. But we did what we could do at the time.

Throughout high school and after graduation, I would constantly be at my friends' houses. We would hang out and be idiots. They hardly came over to my house, but I just figured it was because of this or that. It wasn't until recently that I learned my friends avoided my house because they didn't like going there. They said it was cold. It left them with a terrible feeling. Clearly, they were picking up on the evil that took place in the basement for so many years. That was hard to hear and hard to swallow. All of my friends had these awesome places to hang out, where there was love and warmth. My house wasn't like that.

I can see why they felt that way. Not only were the walls echoing my dad's abuse, but my living space was a reflection of how I felt at the time. And how I felt wasn't good. My mind and spirit were a mess and my room was too. Mess makes it sound cute, but it was beyond a mess. It was the physical representation of my own internal misery. The same can be said about my mom. Hoarding definitely happened. The main areas of the house were filled to the brim with just... stuff. In my own personal space, there would be at least twenty Del Taco wrappers, Wendy's wrappers, Mountain Dew cans, you name it. Same for my car. I was 400 pounds. It takes a lot of food to fuel that weight, so I ate whatever I wanted and never cared about cleaning up after myself. As much as I didn't want to live that way, somehow I could never pick up my clothes or put things away.

It's actually a real thing that when you're depressed, you tend to be messier. In those dark moments of my life, cleanliness was not on my mind. At all. I couldn't have cared less. I didn't care about anything at all. Why would my room matter?

I've come a long way. Messy depression aside, I probably have a healthy amount of untidiness anyway. But I work at being tidier because it's important. Your room and living space affect you whether you realize it or not. It's important that you have pride in your environment because subconsciously it will help you have pride in yourself. Cleaning up after yourself is a baby step in cleaning out the clutter in your mind. Little movements will encourage you to mentally move forward.

One great thing I learned through football is this: Respect your locker. It's important when you're on a team to put your jersey away, to hang up your towel, to make sure that you're taking care of your gear. It's a way to have integrity. Now, I'm not saying locker rooms aren't also disgusting (some of the smells are beyond description), but that is just from the blood, sweat, and tears of the game. My coaches taught me to respect my locker room because how you are off the field affects how you will be on the field. Sports are a mind game. Anything that helps clear your head and steady your thoughts is important for the outcome of a game.

The same thing is true for the locker room that is your home. Clean it up each day. Also, switch things up. Go home and change something in your home. Move your couch. Re-arrange your entire room. Put a picture on the wall. I don't care, just do something. It will help you accept that you're changing and transforming. Changing your environment can change your outlook.

Walking into my house without my dad there felt weird, in a bad way. His controlling presence was gone, but echoes of his words bounced off of the walls. Every nook and cranny of that house invoked a memory involving him. He was that house. We didn't move out until I was in my mid-twenties. Everyone moves forward in their own timing, but I do wish I had had the means to move sooner. It would've helped to not be subconsciously reminded of him when I got a glass of water, or sat on the couch to watch a game, or walked down the stairs to my basement bedroom. That's why I want to help you avoid the mistakes I made. Switch it up. Your living situation does not have to be permanent. Never feel like you're stuck. Start by picking up the trash in your room, just the trash alone, and throwing it away. The next day, put a shirt in the clothes hamper. The day after that, fold your clothes. Little by little, you can clean your room, respect your locker, and, ultimately, respect yourself.

I LIKE TO SAY TO MYSELF

Let's switch things up and clean up.

Chapter 28

Jiggle All the Way

E ven before I was selected to be on the show, I was trying to lose weight. When you're over 400 pounds, working out isn't pretty. It's not like the workout videos where you see guys doing pushups with their muscles flexing and glistening. It's not a yoga instructor, stretching out a strong and slender body to look like a work of art. No, when you're morbidly obese, things are jiggling! You're sweating in places that are not sexy. And the pain on your face, as you gasp for every breath, isn't helping.

The worst part is that there is a small group of people in the world that might make jokes about overweight people working out. We all remember that Chippendales skit on *Saturday Night Live*, right? The one where Chris Farley and Patrick Swayze are both auditioning to be sexy, male dancers. Both are shirtless and both are giving it their all. Chris is severely overweight, while Patrick looks to be chiseled from marble. That skit is hilarious. I laughed. You laughed.

However, the skit reminds me of two things: 1. There will always be that rare person who might laugh at you, and 2. It doesn't matter because confidence is what wins in the end.

But here's what I've really discovered: Most people don't care that you're overweight. In fact, they aren't even looking at you. I got so self-conscious thinking other gym members were judging me, but in reality, they were more concerned about what they looked like. What I've come to discover is that usually the men and women who appear to be the most fit are actually the more self-conscious ones. Really, I'm serious. They are more concerned about what their abs look like than what your jelly-filled gut looks like when it's swinging on that elliptical.

In fact, I would go so far as to say that the people who get the most looks are the fit women. Heidi Powell, one of the hosts of *Extreme Weight Loss*, is the humblest woman in the world. She would never think this or say this, so I'm going to say it for her: She gets more unwanted attention at the gym than an overweight person. I feel sorry for the girls who can't do squats or make gains without having guys constantly objectifying them at the gym.

Most people who go to the gym are insecure about something. Overweight people are worried they will look stupid. But skinny guys worry too. They are afraid that when they can only bench press the bar, with no added weight, that they will embarrass themselves. Old men, skinny girls, juicing body builders—all of them struggle with their own worries at the gym.

All of this has to stop! I've never experienced anyone making fun of me at the gym. I've heard rumors about it happening to others. But I've never actually witnessed anyone being ridiculed. It's so rare that there's really nothing to fear. So don't be afraid to go to the gym. Swallow your pride. You have to throw it out the window. Because when you don't go to the gym, you're only hurting yourself. Trust me. Also, you know what you're doing when you walk into the gym on any given day? You're inspiring somebody because you're in there making an effort to change. If you're bigger than you'd like to be, but you start working out with confidence, you might inspire another person to do the same. The first day you go to the gym, you can help someone else without even realizing it. When you're embarrassed, that's just you, playing games in your head and making another excuse for why you shouldn't go. You have to go back the next day, and the next. You have to embrace the flab! And remember, most of the other gym members are either busy being critical of their own bodies or are happy for you to get healthy!

I LIKE TO SAY TO MYSELF

Embrace the jiggle. No one cares anyway.

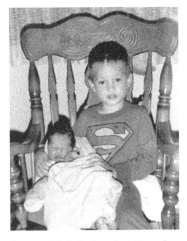 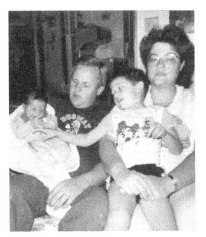

Bruce with baby brother, Brandon   Danny, Janet, Bruce, and baby Brandon

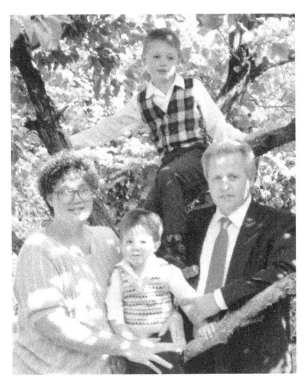

The Pitcher family

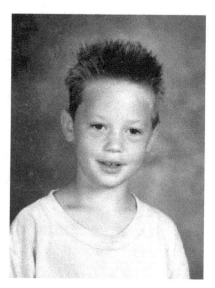

Bruce in second grade, the year his
father's abuse began

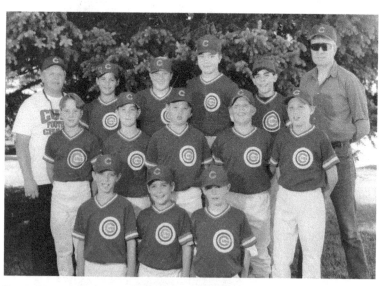

Bruce (center row, center) and his sixth grade Little League baseball team,
coached by his father, Bruce Pitcher (top row, left)

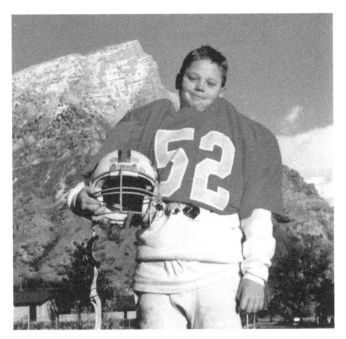

Bruce in seventh grade in his football uniform

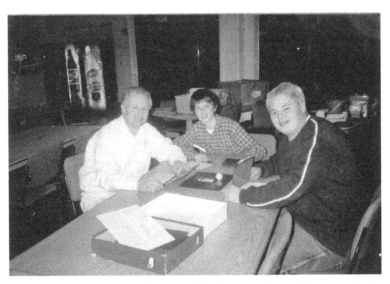

Brandon and Bruce (age 16) on one of their many prison visits to see their father

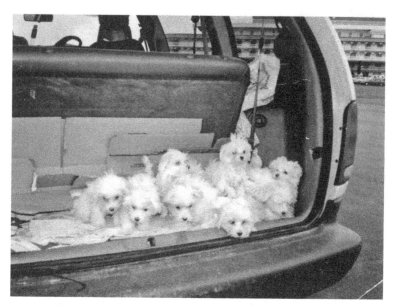

A litter of puppies bred by Bruce and his mother and brother

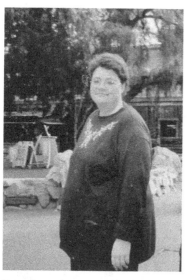

Bruce's mother, Janet, before her weight loss

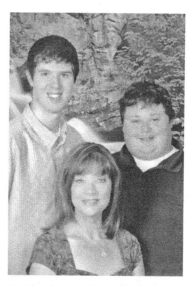

Family photo without Danny Pitcher after Janet's weight loss

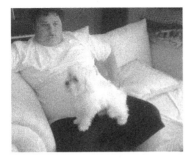

Bruce and one of his dogs, Tex

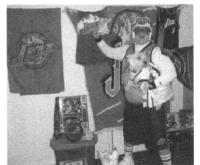

Bruce's Jazz fan contest costume

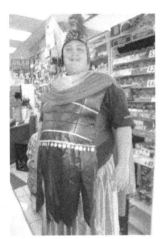

Bruce on Halloween,
working at the gas station

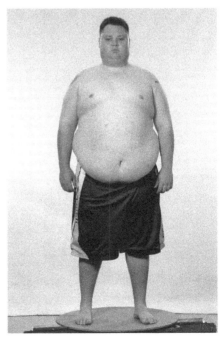

Bruce's official *Extreme Weight Loss*
"before" photograph

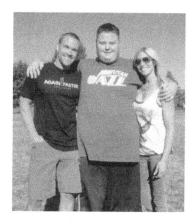

Bruce's arrival in Denver, with
Chris and Heidi Powell

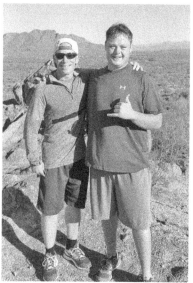

Bruce and J. D. Roth, the producer
who believed in him from the
beginning

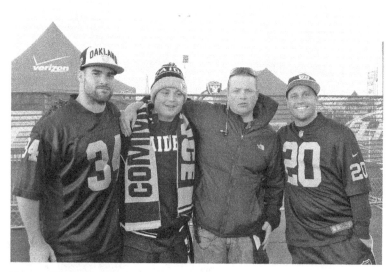

Tommy Hackenbruck, Bruce, Jason Kemp, and Skyler Strong at the
Oakland Raiders visit during Phase 2 of *Extreme Weight Loss*

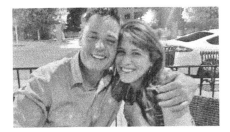

Bruce and Alexa's first photograph together

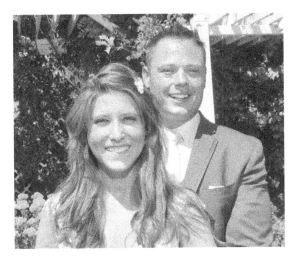

Bruce and Alexa's wedding

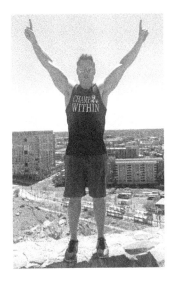

Bruce sporting his shirt for *Champ Within*, the program he started to help others on their weight-loss journey

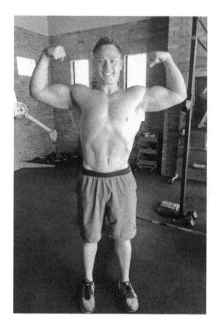

Bruce at 10 percent body fat

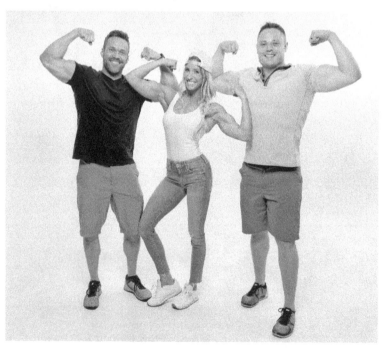

Bruce with Chris and Heidi Powell, who are like family now

Chapter 29

Give 'em Some Sugar

You can't live a perfect day without doing
something for someone who will never be able
to repay you.

—*John Wooden*

've talked a lot about my love for football, but I don't pick favorites when it comes to sports. I love all sports. Also, what else are you going to watch when it's off season for football? John Wooden was one of the greatest, if not the greatest, basketball coach of all time. During his career, he won ten NCAA national championships, seven of them in a row! He was an inspiration on and off the court. He was all about giving to others. It was his belief that if you love others, you get love in return. Coach Wooden had the right idea.

I know from experience that when you are kind and loving to other people it makes the world a better place. Simple as that. Smile and say hi. When you love on others, they love back. Let people know you're loving them. Let them know you're listening to them. When you listen to someone else's trials and help them through, what does it do? It helps you forget your own. When you think about others, you stop thinking about yourself and what's wrong in your life. Seriously, try it. It's pretty hard to be mopey when you're trying to help someone else. And not that this is the goal, but it will all come back to you full circle.

Once, I said "Hi" to someone and it changed my life (I'm not even exaggerating). Before the show, I had my struggles, but I was also still the happy-go-lucky coach, working at the gas station, knocking back Mountain Dew like it was the elixir of life. (About 300 ounces a day, to be exact. That's over 2 gallons! Which is almost 1,300 calories and 350 grams of sugar.) I was just a big dude who liked talking to everyone who came through the door.

One day, Todd Pedersen walked through that door. You probably have never heard of him, but everyone in my town certainly knew him. Todd is one smart guy and all his smarts helped him become pretty dang rich. Years back, he wasn't wealthy or anything, just a normal guy, selling pest control door-to-door. Then he switched to burglar alarms and continued his technique of selling face-to-face, door-to-door. Todd knew the secret early on: When you relate to people on a human level, things just work. His company, now called Vivnt, is this amazing huge company that focuses on home security and energy efficiency. Todd didn't go to college, but he learned by doing. His whole business philosophy was about relating to people by going door-to-door. It's so cool. Anyway, I heard he lived in the area, so when he came in, I wasn't surprised. I wasn't star struck or anything like that. He's such a normal dude that I just treated him like one. I said hi and this and that. He came in often, and we got to talking more and more. It was great, but I didn't think much of it. I talked to all the customers (no offense, Todd).

I was assistant coaching football at the time, but my friend who was coaching little league needed some extra help. I went to the practice and saw Todd. His kid was playing on the team. That's when Todd came up to me and said, "Do you like to bet?" I thought he was talking about sports, so I was stoked. I wanted to know what team and the terms. Sign me up, baby. Still not telling me what the bet was, Todd wanted to know what would hurt me financially. What amount could I bet that would be bad if I lost it, thus motivating me to not lose the bet? He said he didn't care about the money. He just wanted to know what would motivate me. I thought about it and said, "$500." I know it doesn't seem like a lot of money, but at the time, losing $500 would've killed me. He said, "Alright," then laid out the terms of his bet, "If you lose, you give me $500, and if you win, I'll give you $5,000." His bet was that I had to get down to 250 pounds in under a year. Not only was he willing to give me $5,000 if I did it, he also said I could have his personal trainer at my disposal for free! I was pumped. We shook on it, and I got to work.

I started seeing his personal trainer and going to the gym. But I wasn't losing weight that quickly. The employees at the gym tried to help me, but all they would say was, "How's the diet going?" No one mentioned the emotional side of it all. I wanted to crush it and win the bet, but it wasn't looking good.

During that time, I was auditioning for *Extreme Weight Loss* and was selected for the show. I packed my bags and went off to boot camp in Colorado. During the three months I spent at boot camp, I got down to 250 pounds. When I went back home to continue my weight loss, I ran into Todd. He was really proud of me and said, "I believe I owe you some money for a lost bet." I didn't think he should have to pay me.

I lost the weight on the show, and it just didn't feel right, so I told him it would be cool if he hung on to the $5,000. But he's a man true to his word. He gave me the money, and I was floored.

The show gave me more than I could ever afford. But the year I was on the show, I didn't work. I didn't have any money saved before the show, so while my life was evolving and I was moving forward, my bank account was basically at zero. Todd's bet saved me. When you're used to having very little, you also get used to living off of very little for a long time. I knew how to stretch a dollar. I lived off of that $5,000 for as long as I possibly could. Life works that way. You never know where you'll get your next meal sometimes, but God always provides in the weirdest ways.

But Todd's generosity didn't stop there. He genuinely wanted a better life for me so he said, "I'll give you another $5,000 to keep the weight off." I told you he was a smart guy. I like being held accountable, so I took him up on his second bet.

I continued to work hard the rest of the year. The day they filmed the finale for the show, Todd came. I had stayed true to my word and not only kept the weight off, but lost even more too. We all know shows are edited for television. That's cool. But there's something they didn't have enough time to show on TV. During my big reveal, Todd came on stage to give me $5,000 for upholding my end of the bargain. I had less than $100 in my bank account, but I couldn't let him give me the money for a second time. I put my foot down this time and told him to donate the money to Be Your Best. It is this cool organization that helps people get their lives back by overcoming their demons and losing weight. Todd said, "Okay, how about this. I will donate $50,000 to Be Your Best, and I will also give you $5,000 because you won the bet fair and square. Does that sound good?"

I have to brag about Todd Pedersen. He is one of the most generous men I've ever met. He didn't just help the Be Your Best organization and me. He's helped a lot of people. He has made similar bets with people he knows who smoked. He uses the money he has for good. Money doesn't fix everything, but money combined with Todd's caring nature usually does. He totally embraces what John Wooden said. Todd gives, expecting nothing in return.

It's just crazy that all of Todd's impact on my life began because I said hello with a smile. Always remember that. I'm not trying to say that if you say hi to someone you will make a lot of money. Be kind to people because it will brighten their day. You never know who you may be saying hello to or complimenting. They may not improve your life like Todd did for mine. It might be the opposite. Plato said, "Be kind, for everyone you meet is fighting a hard battle."

I LIKE TO SAY TO MYSELF

Be kind. Say hello.

Chapter 30

Get Ready

I didn't want to be 400 pounds. I wasn't okay with being 400 pounds. I just really didn't know how to lose the weight. Everyone tells you the same thing: work out, eat healthy. But without *understanding*, none of it means anything. When I really began to pack on the pounds, I decided to do the only thing I could think of: Go on the TV show *The Biggest Loser*. To me, that was going to solve all of my problems.

Before I auditioned for *Extreme Weight Loss*, I had my sights set on *The Biggest Loser*. I can't tell you how many times I tried to be on that show. I think it was eight times. When the show would come to a city near me, I would go stand in line to be interviewed, with dozens of other overweight hopefuls. My friends helped me film my audition tapes to send in—the whole shebang. I got super close a couple of times too. They would call me back for interviews and background checks. But I never made it on that show. I couldn't understand why at the time, but I get it now. I wasn't ready. It wasn't my time. It's an important lesson to learn.

I thought I was ready because I did try to work out. I would have spurts where I would go to the gym at 6:00 a.m.

and work my butt off. But the problem was, after a workout, I thought I deserved to eat. I would walk out of the gym and there was Del Taco right across the street, like a beacon of fast food goodness. I would get a monster burrito, eat it, and then immediately regret it, thinking, "I'm undoing all I did. What am I doing?" That mindset shows me that I wasn't ready.

The producers for these weight-loss shows genuinely want to help people. They want all of their contestants to be happy, healthy, and whole by the end of it. They hire the best specialists to help them make the decisions about who should be on the show. So much thought goes into it. The producers and specialists at *The Biggest Loser* knew that at that point in my life, I wouldn't succeed. I wasn't in the right place. I was bummed at the time, but now I'm so grateful that they were looking out for me.

A big part of moving forward is being ready to move forward. Don't get me wrong—at a certain point, you have to throw aside all fear and boldly step out, even when you don't feel like it. But you must have the resolve within yourself that it's the right thing to do. Without that, you will fail. Have you ever tried running forward while looking backward? Go outside and try it. Actually, don't try that because you know just as well as I do that you're probably going to get hurt. You'll trip or run into something that will cause you to stumble. It's the same with moving forward mentally and emotionally. When you make the decision to change your life, keep looking forward, never backward. Always shift your focus to your goal. Make a list of why you're doing it and read it every day.

I didn't make it on *The Biggest Loser* because I made the mistake of thinking the show would solve all of my problems.

I had to learn that deep down, it was up to me to do that. I wouldn't have been able to succeed without the tools I acquired on *Extreme Weight Loss*. They saved my life. But at the same time, I wouldn't have succeeded without knowing within myself that I could have a fulfilling life. Both are essential.

Don't beat yourself up for not starting sooner. I did that all the time. Take it from me: Just stop that. Never do that. You can only do what you can do. No moment in your life was or is wasted. It all has a purpose, I promise. The things you may be feeling frustrated with yourself about have already happened, so why dwell on them? You can't change them. Don't feel like a loser or a failure because you weren't ready. It's okay to take your time. Everyone starts at different times. Life can get you down. It's so hard sometimes. It can break your heart. Never feel weak because of that. It happens to all of us. I still have days where I pull the "poor me" card and that's okay, but I try not to stay in that rut.

It's important to remember that your start date is waiting for you. If you want to make a change in your life, and you set your mind on it, the time will come when you will start. You picked up this book and decided to read it. You're already on the right track. Take a moment to decide when it's the right time for you. Take a deep breath and get ready to fly, baby!

I LIKE TO SAY TO MYSELF

Your start day is waiting for you!

Chapter 31

Chris and Heidi

Chris and Heidi Powell take teamwork to another level. Chris was the host of ABC's *Extreme Weight Loss* and Heidi was co-host, working alongside her husband every step of the way. That's just how this dynamic duo goes through life: together. Whether it's workouts, business, personal, or anything in between, these two give it their all, and they make sure to help not only each other, but those around them. They are two of the most genuinely caring people you will ever meet. Their TV personas are their actual personas. Within seconds, you feel the love from both Chris and Heidi.

While they seem to have no trouble making a positive first impression, Chris and Heidi were hesitant when they first saw a hopeful applicant named Bruce Pitcher. After seeing his audition tape, Chris thought to himself, "He's just trying to sell himself." Heidi also had some reservations: "I remember turning to Chris and saying, 'I don't know if that's real.' It was all of his hype." Both Chris and Heidi thought Bruce was faking it. Chris explains, "The first couple interactions I had with Bruce, he was the Bruce that's fired up, ready to go! He hadn't been chosen for the show yet. I knew he was trying to anchor a spot. I've seen it before. That starts to count against them. Sometimes the louder they are, the more it hinders them." After multiple seasons of seeing hundreds, even thousands, of applicants, Chris and Heidi know how many people wanted to be on the show. They got pretty savvy at sniffing out the fake excitement from the real excitement. At first, Chris was worried that Bruce wasn't being authentic. The show is a year long, so for Chris and Heidi, it's like they are married to the people they choose. They are incredibly close to the contestants. It was a big decision for them, and they were having doubts.

But then something happened that caused everything to change. "There's a moment [during the audition process] where everyone sits in a room and they share their stories. We start to dig deeper and get raw. And if they have the courage to share their feelings, their struggles, what happened, that's a real positive for them and for us. Bruce opened his mouth and was so unbelievably real and authentic. At first, you think, 'Here's another loud one.' But then he starts speaking, and it blew my mind. Every word that came out was honest and authentic. It wasn't a sob story, it was him being real. Everyone in the room was blown away. We had to choose him for this opportunity. He was so magnetic!" Chris quickly saw that there was no "pretendo." The same thing happened for Heidi: "You meet in person and you're like, oh my gosh, he's real."

Seeing their relationship with Bruce now, and hearing the things they say, it's hard to believe that initial, and brief, hesitation they had. Now they realize that all of that high energy is just so Bruce. Heidi says she wants to bottle it up and give it to others. Chris is lavish in his praise. Bruce feels like a brother to him. "He loves life. He loves people. He loves connection with people. He's on a level that makes him able to relate to most people. He's courageous. He can read other people like nobody else. He is pretty spot-on with his observations. It's so rare! He's such a gem. He breathes so much life and so much positive spirit into any person he meets."

Heidi also discovered that Bruce has an amazing ability to be a leader in a group. "Bruce is always a leader... not because he wants a power trip, but because people are just drawn to him. You know how people say WWJD? Well, now I feel like a lot of people say WWBD: What would Bruce do?"

Chris and Heidi have been with Bruce through thick and thin. They have been paramount in his success and continue to be a support. Almost all that have watched Bruce make his transformation have said much of it is due to two people: Chris and Heidi Powell. But Chris and Heidi see it the other way around. "I don't think Bruce will ever know the impact he has had on our lives," Heidi says, on the brink of tears, "I say to Bruce, 'You repay us just by being in our lives.'" One word that this power couple uses to describe how they feel to know Bruce is simple, but carries so much weight: "Blessed."

Chapter 32

J. D.

"I wanted him," J. D. says with a heartfelt smile. J. D. Roth is an executive producer and creator of ABC's *Extreme Weight Loss.* That's not the only powerhouse show he's helped create. *The Biggest Loser* is also on his resume, and dozens more. He's the founder and CEO of 3 Ball Productions. But if you're a '90s kid, you may recognize his face from when he was a host on numerous kids' television shows. Even though he has built a successful production empire, J. D. has not let the rat race take away his caring and friendly personality. His red hair and bright blue eyes welcome you with a vibe that makes you feel like you're already friends.

It's apparent that one of the biggest reasons J. D. has been able to produce such hits is because he recognizes potential when a lot of others don't. He has the gift of knowing when to take a chance. He can spot that special something within someone that so often goes unnoticed.

"I had to really stick my neck out for Bruce," J. D. explains. They had narrowed it down to forty potential candidates, Bruce included. When the candidates all left, J. D., Chris and

Heidi, the other producers, and the specialists talked about each of them. It was clear that no one wanted Bruce. "The therapist said it was too risky," J. D. remembers, "and I could see why they said that." Bruce was not at a place yet where he could recognize that what his dad did was wrong. They were worried that when Bruce really delved deep within himself on the show, he might just crash and shut down once he really understood the truth of his story. But J. D. saw it differently. "The only part I can take credit for is looking in his eyes and seeing that he wanted it."

J. D. knew that he was up against almost everyone, so he sat down with Bruce and explained, "Bruce, you're looking at the only person that wants you on the show right now." To prove that Bruce was really fit for the show, J. D. had some guidelines for him. One of them included Bruce losing some weight on his own. Bruce went home and, true to form, did what was asked of him.

Slowly, as they got to know Bruce, the rest of the people involved with the show came to see what J. D. saw all along.

J. D. can't help but laugh now as he remembers what he calls Bruce's infectious enthusiasm. "No one would be working harder. Bruce would scream, 'J. D., this is the best investment you're going to make in your whole life!' Bruce also doesn't just root the other contestants on, he runs to them and drags them across the finish line."

Bruce leaves a positive impression on everyone he meets. But the thing that stays with J. D. the most is actually a quality that Bruce does not possess. "He has no ego. This guy has had incredible darkness. Along the way, he thought he knew what love was and he didn't. He has this huge capacity for love for someone who was loved so inappropriately.

He is doing the exact opposite of what was expected of him. He engages in the most emotional intimacy he can. He's not afraid to put himself out there."

ABC's *Extreme Weight Loss* is not just a gimmick. J. D. explained the stats. "Normally, people that lose 100 pounds or more have a 5 percent success rate of keeping it off. For shows like *Extreme Weight Loss* and *The Biggest Loser*, it's ten times that." Fifty percent of their contestants keep the weight off. Bruce is within that 50 percent because of his own determination and the ability of the show to encourage him and help him grow.

Bruce had another natural quality that J. D. could see from the get-go: "He didn't feel sorry for himself." Throughout the audition process and the taping, Bruce never played the victim. It was key to his success. "After what he's been through, to have that frame of mind is incredible. He doesn't wallow in the bad things that happened. He just says, 'I'm going to have the best attitude of anyone you've ever met.' That's the foundation of who he is."

J. D. ends with one final observation, "Bruce's dad took so much from him. But there was one thing his dad couldn't abuse out of Bruce: his kindness. To me, that's incredible."

Chapter 33

Hey... You

Chris and Heidi Powell are superheroes here on earth. I have trouble expressing how much they changed my life and how much they mean to me. I cry every time I think about it. Every. Damn. Time.

Being a TV host sometimes carries with it a negative image about your personality. A host seems robotic and potentially cold when the cameras are off. Chris and Heidi are nothing like that. They are just as genuine on the screen as they are off. They have become celebrities in the world's eyes, but to me, they are just my best friends and people I consider family. You would think that after the show they might move on and leave me in the dust. They are busy people, after all. I probably would have understood if they didn't have time. But they have been there for me from day one of the show to day one after the show, and every day since. I can call them up any time—day or night—and they are there for me. I share with them my triumphs, and they help me carry my failures without hesitation.

The way they treat me is so different from the way my own dad did. My dad was never a dad to me. He never taught me how to be a man. I don't mean a tough, macho, manly man. I just mean the type of guy that people think, "That's a good man." That's where Chris and Heidi come in. Chris supports his wife and kids. He provides for them financially and loves on them like nobody's business. He makes sure to put his family first. Even when he's improving himself, he's doing it for them. That's a real man to me. Chris taught me that.

The Powells have gone above and beyond for me. I never feel like I deserve their kindness and love, but they insist that I stop saying that. Because my life was so altered by my dad, by the time I was thirty, I had never even had a bank account. Heidi helped me open my own bank account. They helped me buy my first car. They coached me on how to get out of debt.

I could go on and on about them. But one small memory has really stuck with me. It's something I learned from them, and something I hope you can take with you as well.

The audition process for *Extreme Weight Loss* is long and tedious. Chris, Heidi, and all of the other producers evaluate hundreds of people who are hoping to be on the show. The Powells and producers take great care and spend a long time sifting through the hopefuls and picking contestants they think will benefit from the show. They bring in the help of therapists and other specialists to make sure each person is ready for the experience. First there are auditions. Then there are the audition tapes. Then the phone interviews—so many phone interviews. Then they narrow it down to around forty potential candidates. They fly them out. Even more interviews, background checks, and physicals, and then workouts begin.

When all of us hopefuls were gathered in a room, I remember that Chris and Heidi already knew all of us by name and even knew pieces of our lives. They had taken the time to learn about each and every one of us before they even met us. That they remembered our names stood out to me.

Losing the weight and becoming fit is not just about looking like a better person; it's about *becoming* a better person. The benefit of having a trimmer physique is an added bonus. On this path of shedding pounds, you'll find that the true transformation happens on the inside. Your heart becomes better looking.

I like to do exercises for my heart. The best way to gain a fuller heart is to use it every day. Just like any other muscle, when you don't exercise your heart, it begins to atrophy, which makes it harder to use, which makes it atrophy even worse, on and on, worse and worse, until you're 400 pounds and you find it difficult to even talk to another person.

Research has found that one of the words we like hearing the most is our own name. It's where we place our entire identity. It's ours. And when someone takes the time to remember it, it tells us that they cared enough to store such an important part of who we are. Chris and Heidi understand that.

There was a time when I didn't like my name: Bruce Pitcher. The first part was alright, but the last part was the part that bugged me. I hated that my last name was attached to the last name of my abuser. I disliked it so much that I wanted to change it. I always loved Batman and John Wayne, so I thought I would change it to Bruce Wayne. He was a superhero—something I wanted to be. I wanted nothing more than to fly away from all of that darkness with my cape behind me.

But I realized that I couldn't run from my past. It's what made me who I am today. My name—my full name—is who

I am. It carries the trials and the trauma, but it also is my moniker for overcoming all of that. My dad doesn't own me anymore. He is not where I find my worth. I am not Danny Pitcher. I'm Bruce Pitcher. We may share a last name, but we are completely different people.

Bruce Pitcher is a guy who has been through living hell and made it out. Like steel forged in the fire, Bruce Pitcher has become stronger through the raging flames of his life. I not only like my name now, I love it. I love Bruce Pitcher.

Something you can do that will exercise your heart and keep your spirit healthy is to remember someone's name. It doesn't require any physical activity. You don't have to cut carbs to achieve it, but it will help you on your journey toward a new you. Taking the time and energy to remember one word as simple as a name will actually help you lose weight.

I LIKE TO SAY TO MYSELF

Make someone's day.
Remember their name.

Chapter 34

The Beginning

I was twenty-nine years old when my life would be forever changed. All of the auditions were done. The producers sent us back home while they decided who they would pick. Typical me, I just tried not to think about it.

The way the show works is that Chris shows up to surprise the contestant and tell them they have been chosen to participate in the greatest experience of their life. Crew from the show had come to Utah once before to get some footage. It was all a part of the process. They told me and the other hopefuls that cameras would probably show up again at some point. However, they said not to get our hopes up about Chris showing up. I know what you're thinking—if cameras are there, Chris is going to be there. But that wasn't the case. All of us hopeful contestants were calling and texting each other. I got the word that a camera crew was with this guy I met during auditions, and Chris never showed up. That guy didn't ever get picked for the show. When I heard that, I was worried. I didn't know whether it would work out or not. I had made it pretty far a couple of times for *The Biggest Loser* and failed to get on the show, so I thought maybe that would happen again.

So one day I was working out in the gym with the crew filming me. It was nerve-wracking. I had been working out for a while and still no sign of Chris. I thought it was all over, and I for sure thought he wasn't going to show up. Then, I'll never forget it... I hear this voice, "Bruce! Who's the man?" I knew instantly it was Chris. Greatest moment of my life! Chris said, "I choose you for the transformation of your life." It was the opportunity of a lifetime. I was so thankful. I was all sweaty from working out, but I didn't care. I hugged Chris probably a little too hard. I've never been so happy. I definitely started crying. And just like that, I was going to be on season four of ABC's *Extreme Weight Loss*.

That was just the beginning. They flew me out to Colorado to start Phase 1 of my transformation at the University of Colorado Anschutz Health and Wellness Center. It's one of the top ten facilities in the world for treating obesity. Walking into the Anschutz Center was like walking into something you never knew existed. You got medical stuff, steam room, pool—all these great things. It's like, "Wow! If you can't succeed here, I don't know what to tell ya." They knew on the show to work on your body, but also to work on your heart. The heart was what would always break me. I liked how the process worked because I wasn't going to lack motivation on the workouts; it would be the mental stuff that I would have to work hardest on.

Something else really special happened the first day I showed up in Colorado: I got to be with Heidi Powell, one-on-one, for a couple of days. Chris isn't the only fit person in their household. Heidi is one very fit woman! But more importantly, she is one tuned-in person. She cares deeply about each and every person she comes in contact with, especially the ones she's trying to help. She is a workout guru and has dedicated her life to learning the best techniques in order to help others. All of the contestants live together and train together, but none of them were there yet, so she and I got this amazing time to ourselves to bond and start off right.

Heidi has a background similar to mine, so we were able to connect instantly on a level that I don't share with a lot of people. She was raised LDS; her brothers had gone on missions. Plus, Heidi always just made me feel loved. I didn't have to be somebody to her, I could just be myself and she liked me.

Life is one big surprise like that. You never know when something big is coming or if it's coming. But trust me, your own special moments will come. Before this happened, I was for sure in the lowest part of my life. I didn't want to be alive. I couldn't see any way out, and I thought I would die in such a dark place. But there are always good things just around the corner. When you're in the darkness, it's hard to remember that good things are coming, but they are. Believe that. Wonderful things will come into your life in an instant and change you for the better, forever.

I LIKE TO SAY TO MYSELF

Good surprises are ahead!

Chapter 35

Know Your Why

The whole auditioning process for *Extreme Weight Loss* was long. I would be lying if I didn't say that through it all, I kept imagining what it would be like to be on the show. But when I officially was selected and flew out to Colorado, I really didn't know what to expect. I had no idea what was in store for me. Here's a little behind the scenes look for you.

A day in the week of *Extreme* boot camp went a little something like this: First of all, there is this large production crew that you never see on camera. They are the ones responsible for making sure everything runs smoothly. The camera guys, the sound guys, the production assistants, the producers, and everyone in between do not get enough credit for all they do. The night before, they would give us a schedule for the next day. Typically, we would wake up around 6:00 a.m. and eat breakfast within thirty minutes of waking up. We would get ready and wait for the two cast vans to show up. The cast coordinators would load the contestants in the van to take us to a place to work out. There were sixteen of us, all 400-plus-pound people.

We would go to a football field or somewhere like that. Then came the shredder: This was two hours of the most intense cardio you can imagine. It would include running around a track, up and down bleachers, doing Indian runs, and then playing a game of some sort. At first, the shredders were nearly impossible for most of the contestants. Carrying around an extra 200 pounds is no easy feat when you're sprinting 50 yards. Chris and Heidi were usually there to take us through these workouts, which was a huge motivator.

After the shredder, we would all go home and eat a snack and take a little break. But before long it was time for another workout. The vans and the coordinators would show up again and take us to a CrossFit class (with Alex Takacs and Caleb Sommer of Project Rise Fitness). I flippin' loved the CrossFit sections and I still do. It's totally my kind of working out. Those workouts were more about resistance and all-around muscle building.

We would come home and eat a healthy lunch. It's super important to properly fuel your body when so much physical activity is happening. Then we got to rest a little more, hang out, whatever. After lunch, we were taken to the Anschutz Health and Wellness Center for mindset classes, to help with the mental stuff. They would teach us everything—from the science behind your metabolism to how to shop for groceries and the psychology behind it. They would take our stats and make sure we were all healthy.

After that, we went back home and had "Cardio Fun Time." All that meant was that we could do whatever we wanted, as long as we weren't sitting around. We could go on a walk, swim in the pool or Jacuzzi, play some basketball—it just had to be active. No problem for me there. I've always been an active guy and I love sports.

After that, we had dinner. I always loved the evenings at the house because we would just laugh and hang out. There is a lot of bonding that happens when you're together 24/7. But it wasn't just about being around each other all the time, it was sharing the same life-changing experience with another human being. That's something that you can't describe.

Then we would go to bed. Getting enough sleep is a big component of shedding the weight. Trust me, it wasn't hard to fall asleep after the days we had.

And that was the schedule during the week. They would switch up the workouts, but the basic structure remained. Toward the end of the week, we usually had an activity to do together, like bowling or a movie. Also, once a week, I would go to counseling to learn how to process everything that happened with my dad.

Sundays were our rest days. Our bodies needed to heal and recover after putting in so much hard work. And we were allowed a reset meal. This was a meal in which we were allowed to eat whatever we wanted. Something that has helped me with my weight loss is to not make any food off limits forever. Meaning, there are foods to avoid on a regular basis, but I don't cut them out completely. If I were to swear off donuts for the rest of my life, it would just make me think about donuts and want them more. Then, if I ate a donut, I might just eat two or three because I was craving them so much. I would fall off the wagon entirely. But if I allow myself a reset meal, or indulgence meal, it helps me with my cravings. On Sundays, we weren't allowed to eat whatever we wanted all day, just for one meal.

I loved how relaxing Sundays were. However, Sundays were also our weigh-in days, so a lot of my friends in the house didn't feel very restful. Getting weighed is stressful.

But after several weeks of consistently losing, you start gaining confidence. You start realizing the program is working and that you're achieving your dreams. When we did our weigh-ins, they had us step on the scale backward. They wouldn't tell you what it said right there. They would take you to another room, sit you down, and then tell you. All of that "suspense and drama" was better for television, but it also made it feel more important to me personally. Let's say you gained that week. That usually meant you would meet with Chris. One-on-ones with Chris were always helpful when you were struggling. Or, maybe you reached a milestone in your weight loss, like you lost 100 pounds, then they would film a celebratory thing.

The other thing I learned about how they filmed was that they didn't film you every second of every day. They would say in advance when the camera crew would be there. If they wanted to film you alone, or with Chris and Heidi, they would usually do it in the morning because sunrise is the best light. That meant that we would do our shredder in the afternoon instead of the morning on those days. They would mic you for interviews, but if it was B roll (footage that doesn't have dialogue), they wouldn't need to because they weren't going to be using sound. That was helpful because sometimes they would mic you during workouts and it felt awkward to have a sound pack attached while you were doing burpees, for example.

The three months we spent in Phase 1 were full of hard work and dedication. The focus was on teaching us how to be healthy and then showing us how to apply what they taught us. I really felt pumped up by all the workouts. The workout part was challenging, but not in a mental way for me. It was challenging physically because I was swinging around a lot of extra weight. The harder part was learning all the little things, like how to shop, how to cook, how to think about everything.

While the schedule seemed really full every day, after a while, I have to admit, it got boring at times. We didn't have cable. We did have internet, so we would hook up our computers to the TV screen so we could watch the games or a movie or something. There was a clubhouse that we would hang out in. We were allowed to have our phones and call people. But we absolutely could NOT send pictures. I thought it was fun to keep how much weight I had lost a secret. It made the ninety-day reveal to friends and family that much more fun. But you do miss the people you left back home. You do have moments where it's not just hunky-dory. I have to admit that I never really liked when we went on hikes. I'm all for people liking hiking, but for me, it's like kryptonite. But when I started to have moments that left me feeling like I was running out of steam, I remembered my "why."

Something they asked me early on was, "Why do you want to be on the show?" In the beginning, I thought my why was because I wanted to look good. That's how I would answer when I tried out for *The Biggest Loser.* I didn't understand it at all. I just thought, "Well, I just want to be healthy and feel good about myself." That answer didn't get me very far in the auditioning process. The more I went along, the more I realized that I was afraid to admit my real "why" because the truth gets me so emotional. The show helped me see that I wanted to lose weight because I wanted to be loved. My why has always been love.

At my first workout with Chris at Red Rocks Amphitheater, he stripped away all of the invisible walls I had built around me. He broke me down and that's when I knew my why 100 percent. After I knew what it was, it drove me. But I was also being fed love and support through the show. It was a win-win.

When days would get boring or hard (or we went on a hike), I would always come back to why I was doing it. When I remembered what was driving me, it gave me the strength to keep going. I encourage you to find your why. Once I was able to say I was losing weight because I wanted to feel loved, the weight just melted off. And in a wonderful surprise, the show gave me love. Coming back to your why is a way to keep your integrity. And integrity will always be the best kind of fuel.

If you don't know why you're doing something, or you're coming up with a weak answer in your mind like I was, it's nearly impossible to change your life. Dig down deep. Put in the work to figure out what is driving you. It'll pay off in the end, I promise.

I LIKE TO SAY TO MYSELF

Know your why.

Chapter 36

Inheritance vs. Choice

I already mentioned that my dad came from money. His parents (my grandparents) have allotted inheritance money to all their children. However, after I came forward with the truth about how my dad sexually abused me for six years, my grandparents wrote my mom, Brandon, and me out of their will. I love my grandparents, but they are most likely under that manipulative spellbinding that my dad does so well. They believe my dad's lies and think I'm the one lying. When I think about it that way, it makes sense that they wouldn't want me or any of my immediate family to receive any inheritance. It's okay, though. It's never bothered me that much. Their actions have taught me a valuable lesson: Inheritance should never be expected because it isn't a given. This lesson has helped me in all areas of my life, especially when I apply it to attitude. You don't inherit your attitude, it isn't a given. You choose your attitude.

I never struggled with a bad attitude when it came to working out, but I'll admit that I wasn't always happy to give up a lot of foods I loved. Before the show, there were no limits to my eating. When I went out to eat, I would throw down a giant nacho appetizer by myself, then I would get a massive burrito, and I'd wash the whole thing down with soda that would be refilled multiple times throughout the meal. I ate Reese's Pieces like they were going out of business. I had fast food all the time. I would spend at least fifteen to twenty dollars at Wendy's: a classic triple, two junior bacon cheeseburgers, some chicken nuggets, maybe some fries, and the largest soda I could order. But my downfall was Mountain Dew. I drank it like it was water. I was drinking at least three gallons of it a day. Working at the gas station meant that I had an unlimited supply.

When I started the show, my diet did a complete 180. We followed a carb-cycling diet that Chris and Heidi Powell had come up with (if you want to learn more about it, or try it yourself, check out their app: Transform with Chris and Heidi). Basically, you do four days of high carbs, two days of low carbs, and one day off. On high carb days, you eat 280–300 grams of good carbs like brown rice, potatoes, fruit, fat free popcorn, whole grain tortillas, things like that. On low carb days, you eat 60 grams of carbs for the day. Obviously, it was always low fat, but never *no* fat. Fat is important in a diet if you eat the right amount. On high carb days, we would do lower fat, about 40 grams. On low carb days, we would do a little more fat, about 90–100 grams. While good fats were okay, sugar was almost entirely cut out. We could occasionally have sugar-free foods but that was it. For protein, guys got four to six ounces of protein per meal and the women got three to four ounces per meal. We kept track of all of this in a food log that we had to fill out religiously. If we were doing it right, weigh-ins on Sundays were successful.

We were given a stipend to buy groceries and would usually go out once or twice a week to stock up. I would go with my roommates, Jayce, Rod, and David. We called ourselves the four horsemen. I love these dudes. I mean it. We were a tight group that was always together. We all came from different places, but the show connected us. Jayce was a Nashville songwriter. Rod was a drama teacher. David was a chef from Missouri. It was nice having David in the house because he could whip up some really good (and healthy) meals. He would keep to the program but create things you liked to eat, so we had fun with the menus.

The cheat meal on Sundays really helped with the cravings. Plus, I was so excited and motivated. I just wanted to be successful, so I followed the program. In the beginning, the first little bit, when you are losing weight, it's the best feeling in the world. That feeling really kept me going.

But as good as David was and as dedicated as I felt, there were times when I really missed my old diet. It sounds crazy because how could I miss something that made me feel terrible and caused me to gain so much weight? Those old foods were comforts to me and that's the truth. I never wavered from the new eating program they taught us, but I had to work at not being upset about following it. And that's when I came back to this idea of choosing your attitude over inheriting it.

The meal plan was really hard at first. I could've had a bad attitude about it. But any time I got close to resenting the lean meats and lack of soda, I remembered how thankful I was to be on the show and to be learning how to take care of myself. I thought about how grateful I was for the opportunity. My attitude was positive. I wasn't given that mindset. It wasn't an inheritance to be expected. It was something I chose.

Choosing to focus on the good and choosing to have a good attitude was one of the keys to my success on the show and in life. At other times in my life, before the show, I had a bad attitude. I didn't know how to process what my dad did to me. I didn't know how to cope with him being gone. So I got depressed. That's understandable, right? I could've lived with that attitude forever. I learned on the show that a hopeful outlook isn't given to you, but if you can choose to have it, it will give you more than you ever imagined. Choosing a good attitude will give you peace under the most difficult circumstances.

I LIKE TO SAY TO MYSELF

You don't inherit your attitude,
you choose it.

Chapter 37

Caleb and Alex

When Caleb Sommer (owner of Project Rise Fitness in Denver, Colorado) got the call that *Extreme Weight Loss* wanted to use his facilities for their contestants, he was floored. Caleb is a three-time CrossFit Games competitor, and he knew he had the skills and equipment to help, but he didn't know what to expect. He enlisted the help of his right-hand man, Alex Takacs, to help tailor workouts for the contestants. "It was an amazing opportunity. But it was a massive puzzle," Alex confesses. Caleb adds that the hardest part was helping the contestants overcome the emotional and mental obstacles: "We got them basically on day one. They were 400 pounds. They didn't want to be there. They complained constantly. As it is with quitting any addiction, it's really hard to start. They were fighting and trying to overcome some serious demons." Caleb and Alex decided to implement their shared philosophy when it comes to training others: Figure out what motivates each individual.

Caleb and Alex set out to create workouts that were achievable and would be appropriate for the contestants' abilities.

"These guys simply just wanted to love themselves again. It took on a new meaning when we were programming and creating their workouts. I found myself trying to use movements that were accessible. And ones that would have a low barrier, so they would be able to accomplish the movement and eventually go past the barrier," Alex explains. The guys knew that if the contestants failed at the workouts, they might consider it one more in a long list of failures. They wanted the contestants to feel like they were winning at something.

Caleb and Alex knew the contestants wanted to lose weight, but many had a bad attitude at the start. Caleb explains, "In the beginning, it was hard to figure out how to motivate them. They would always complain they had an injury, anything to get out of doing the workout." However, there were a few that didn't seem to have the same mindset. "David, Rod, and Bruce were three positive exceptions that were head and shoulders above the rest in the beginning. But Bruce was above them all. So we instantly latched on to Bruce to help us encourage the others, because his energy level was so high. His weight didn't stop his energy level. He was pumped on life. It was really easy to connect with him. I never noticed a bad day. He would get frustrated with himself when his body wouldn't do what his mind wanted to. He was a different animal because he wouldn't stop. The others had trouble getting out of their comfort zones. Not the same with Bruce."

Alex saw that while some of the contestants needed a little more encouragement or tenderness to get started, "Bruce was always ready to slay the dragon and constantly strike." And while Bruce may have started on a high, Caleb observed how all the contestants got there eventually too. "They all had their own timeline for overcoming that mental side. Every single one of them, by the time the year was over, overcame it mentally." Both guys loved watching the life-changing improvements the contestants made.

Caleb and Alex feel honored to have been a part of all these transformations. They loved watching and helping each individual person, especially Bruce. "There are some rare opportunities where you get to look at someone's life and see the stars align for them. When Bruce stepped out of the fear and discomfort of being the larger Bruce, you just got to see the dominos fall perfectly. He was on this upward trajectory all the time. He was hitting all his numbers. Once Bruce gained the tools from the show, he was able to understand that this journey was becoming bigger than himself. He went from this guy that was all about hitting his numbers to this guy that understood that his purpose was greater than losing his weight. It drove him further. He was always searching for more purpose. That's what makes him such a great motivator because he knows that's his purpose. He wants to help people." Caleb adds, "We didn't have to motivate Bruce. We had to motivate almost every other person, but not Bruce. He would come into the gym, wearing these giant, oversized t-shirts. His belly was so large that it made him lean back a little. And he would be yelling, throwing his hands up, saying 'Let's do this!' He was just pumped up every single day. That stood out like crazy to me and will always stay with me."

Alex recalls that "when Bruce would walk into the gym, he would bring an entire new energy. Seeing Bruce every day, it is the same way your dog greets you at the door. He's happy you're there and can't wait to just be with you. Seeing that immense appreciation and gratitude to just be alive is truly life-changing. You wouldn't have to work out or even talk to him that much, you could just tell Bruce was grateful to be there with you. Bruce showed me personally that your attitude is a choice... you're in control."

Chapter 38

Never Give Up

It's okay to feel hopeless sometimes, but it's also important that you never give up. It's a strange dichotomy. But what I mean is that you have to find a balance. You can take mental sick days. You can just not be feeling it, but deep down—deep, deep down—you have to keep moving forward. You have to know within your heart that you matter. Because when you feel valuable, that's the fuel to keep you going when things don't go the way you planned.

I know things didn't always go how I planned. Getting selected for the show felt like winning the lottery. My whole life was changing so fast, and everything was getting better. Now I had Chris and Heidi, special trainers, doctors, dieticians, producers—everyone was there to help me. It was hard work, but I was in heaven. I was losing weight every single week. I set records on the show. All of my dreams were coming true. But two months into boot camp, all of that would change.

On the show, all of the contestants spend the first three months in Colorado at the Anschutz Center. It's an intense—and condensed—time of training and coaching to help prepare you for the rest of the year. You eat, sleep, and breathe one idea all day long: Get healthy.

One day, all of us were in the pool for a fun, group exercise. We were playing Sharks and Minnows. I'm a competitive guy, so I probably took the game a little too seriously. My competitiveness, combined with my sheer determination, made me a little overzealous. I went under water and kicked off the wall as hard as I could. Out of nowhere, I slammed into something head first. It was so hard. Oh my heck, I felt so dazed. I thought it must've been someone's knee. I surfaced and looked around to see who it was. Someone's knee had to be killing them, but there was no one. I had an instant headache, but I carried on anyway. I figured, well, I got hit in the head. It's bound to hurt. That night, my headache was worse, but I decided to sleep it off.

The next morning, they took us all to an amusement park. I still had a headache and felt dizzy, but I wasn't about to miss out on the fun. No joke, we went on a ride called the Mind Eraser. I know you're probably cringing at this point, but yes, I went on the ride. It's the type of ride where your legs are dangling, and you have a harness that goes over your shoulders with your head resting in between the padded rods. When the ride began, all "resting" and "padding" went out the window, as my head was rattled between the rods of the harness like a ball in a pinball machine. When I got off, I was not doing too hot. My head hurt worse than ever, and my world was spinning. However, I like to stay positive, so I chalked it up to my age. The last time I went on a roller coaster, I was a lot younger. Maybe I was too old for these types of shenanigans now. Apparently, that thought didn't stick too well in my altered state because... I got on the ride again.

After that second round on the Mind Eraser, I was done. I couldn't do anything more at the amusement park. I couldn't leave, so I just sat down and tried not to focus on the fact that my head felt ready to explode.

I know you're cringing. I know you're thinking that, surely, I went to the doctor at this point. That would've been the wise thing to do, but I was a guy with, most likely, a brain injury, so I cut myself some slack for not doing anything.

No doctor that day. The next morning was our Sunday Funday. The contestants and I were hanging out at the house. At this point, my friends were starting to notice that I was acting funny. I kept telling Jayce to take my shirt off. Everyone, including Jayce, informed me that Jayce was not wearing my shirt. But that's not what I saw. Jayce was wearing my shirt, and it was really bugging me. To this day, I would swear on my life that he was wearing my shirt. I began throwing up that day and finally—finally!—as soon as the show found out, they got me to go to the doctor.

As you probably guessed by now, I had a severe concussion. But that wasn't the worst part. I was told that I couldn't work out for at least a month. I can't describe how devastating this news was to me. I had been making so many gains. I was cruising. But if they took physical activity away from me, I knew all that would change. How was I going to lose weight if I couldn't burn calories?

The last month of boot camp I had to just sit everything out. It sucked. I've always been a team player, but now I had to sit on the sidelines. I decided to take matters into my own hands and work out anyway. I would sneak out to get a little run in or lift some weights, but someone from the show caught me. From that point on, they began to monitor me because I wasn't following doctor's orders. I can see now why they would do that, but in the moment, all I cared about was doing what I went there to do.

The three months of Phase 1 were up, and it was time to go home and practice all of the things I had learned. However, I still couldn't work out. The doctor said I wasn't allowed to resume normal training until I went a week without having symptoms. (Keep in mind, this whole time I still had headaches and dizziness.) It took another month at home before I was symptom-free. That was two whole months that I didn't lift one dumbbell, didn't do one burpee, and didn't elevate my heart rate. Heidi called my trainers at home and really broke it down, "He's going to say he's fine, but he's not. You have to watch him like a hawk." I laugh thinking about it now. I was very resistant to the idea of not working out!

I could've given up. I had a brain injury. But I didn't. I dedicated myself to eating clean and sorting out my emotional health. I exercised my heart by telling myself every day that I would keep moving forward, no matter the setback. I wasn't going to let this get in the way of accomplishing my goal.

In the end, all of the discipline and hard work paid off. I didn't gain any weight like I feared. I lost weight. I lost weight almost every week for eight weeks without working out. I didn't give in to an "impossible" situation because I refused to believe that it was impossible. It was a huge disappointment, sure, but it was nothing I couldn't overcome if I kept trying.

I LIKE TO SAY TO MYSELF

A setback can be a step up.

Chapter 39

Holly and Donielle

"He was the absolute *worst*! You can quote me on that," Dr. Holly Wyatt laughs as she describes how rebellious Bruce was after his concussion. She should know. Dr. Wyatt, who prefers to be referred to as Dr. Holly, is a physician, and is one of the leaders at the Anschutz Health and Wellness Center. She coauthored the book *State of Slim,* revealing how Coloradans get and stay slim. Because of her extensive research in clinical weight-loss studies, *Extreme Weight Loss* appointed her to give medical clearance to all the contestants on the show, as well as to oversee all of their medical stats during Phase 1.

Her right-hand woman was Donielle Montoya, who jokes that she was the contestants' mom away from home. Together, the women would help the contestants if they were sick, injured, or anything in between. They specially tailored programs to fit the needs of each contestant. And when it came to Bruce, they had no problem getting him to work out. However, it was another story when they tried to get him to stop working out because of his concussion. "I would have to go into the gym almost every day and tell him to stop,"

Donielle says. She says Bruce would use every trick in the book to evade her, often changing his shirt so she wouldn't think he was still in the gym. "He would even hide behind things so I wouldn't see him… which obviously didn't work."

But through it all, the colleagues couldn't help but be struck by the light that emanates from Bruce's heart. Dr. Holly explains how the Anschutz Center helps people on their weight-loss journey: "The idea is that everything is under one roof—expertise in physical fitness, in diet, body composition measurement, research and clinical programs—all going on side-by-side. We offer cooking demos, teaching people how to cook. There's a full gym. And it's all in one place. We have all the tools to match people in what they need."

For example, Dr. Holly discovered that Bruce needed a little extra help in the nutrition department. The center is equipped with a mini grocery store to help contestants learn how to shop. They were also sensitive to Bruce's past, "Bruce got extra counseling… We felt like he needed psychological counseling." However, Dr. Holly explains that, even given his blind spots in nutrition and a few other areas, Bruce came in with a different attitude than the rest. "Sometimes people start in the 'it's-not-fair stage,' like a kid with a temper tantrum: 'It's not fair that I'm struggling with my weight.' You have to get past that phase to get to true change. Bruce was past that. He had a great attitude. In spite of what happened to him, he had a positive mindset. He believed that he could change things. He just needed some help. He was always firing people up and ready to go. He was the first one to do things. Bruce was never about drama. He was never about all the things he couldn't do. He just always gave 110 percent."

Both women say that Bruce was always there for his fellow contestants. One of Donielle's favorite stories to tell about

Bruce when he was on the show is when one of Bruce's room-mates, David, was in the hospital and wanted to stay on track with his eating, so he asked Bruce to bring him some food. Ever faithful and dedicated, Bruce brought a frozen turkey, a can of green beans, and a raw potato. Bruce dutifully handed off the items to Donielle and went on his way. Donielle stared incredulously at the items and thought, "What is David going to do with these in the hospital?" Donielle says that Bruce's impractical but kindhearted act remains a fond memory for everyone on the show.

Donielle had a strong maternal instinct when it came to Bruce: "You just love the kid. He's infectious. There's some-thing about him, you don't know what it is. You just want to help him. You just want to do that as another mother." Donielle was the person the contestants would call late at night when something was wrong, or any time throughout the day. She was so on the pulse when it came to Bruce that "he could just give me a look and I would know what he needed."

After the show was over, Bruce stayed in Colorado to help the next season, but he had no place to live. True to her motherly nature, Donielle, a mother of six children, three of whom were still living at home, opened up her home to the new, and healthier, Bruce. "Bruce had a special relationship with my husband." Recognizing that Bruce had missed out on a lot when it came to a father figure, Donielle's husband was more than happy to fill in. "One time, around Christmas, my husband was wrapping presents. Bruce went and got the presents he needed wrapped and brought them to my hus-band as if to say, 'Can you wrap these too?' But instead, my husband taught Bruce to wrap presents." Bruce also became heavily involved with Dr. Holly's Destination Boot Camp, a twelve-week program to help people kick-start their weight-loss journey.

Both Dr. Holly and Donielle talk about Bruce as family. "You immediately love him. Like a little brother," Dr. Holly says affectionately. Donielle is certain that "Bruce will always be a part of our family."

Chapter 40

Fear

If you know the enemy and know yourself,
you need not fear the result of a hundred battles.
If you know yourself but not the enemy, for every
victory gained you will also suffer defeat.
If you know neither the enemy nor yourself,
you will succumb in every battle.

—*Sun Tzu*, The Art of War

A big part of the process on the show was counseling. I couldn't get physically healthy until I was mentally healthy. It took me a while because, for a long time, I didn't know who the enemy was. I never even thought I had an enemy. I attributed all my negative feelings to my own failures as a person.

Brilliant is a strange word to use to describe a terrible thing. The word brilliant sounds like a good thing. But I've learned over the years that there is a mastery and brilliance in evil things too, as sad as that is. My dad was brilliant at manipulating. He was brilliant at grooming victims. But the difference between my dad's brilliance and the brilliance of someone else is that my dad's brilliance doesn't make him a good person. It's not something you want to be good at. It's not something to be praised for. I'm not praising him or tipping my hat. I just want to describe him the way he was.

What did my dad do that was so brilliant? He made his victims believe that he wasn't the enemy. He made me believe he wasn't the enemy. His actions were sadistic. He held positions of power and trust in these kids' lives, and he used that to teach them a lie.

His most powerful position was as a father. A son looks up to his dad. Without doing anything, the moment you become a dad, you also become your child's hero. Just the name tag makes you Superman in his eyes. My dad abused this idea. He twisted his evil actions into something that seemed good to his victims, including me. By making us believe everything was normal and great, we became completely unable to identify our attacker. Like Sun Tzu said, if you don't know who the enemy is, you will suffer defeat half the time.

But it goes further than that. My dad's conditioning did something else. Slowly, over time, I forgot who I was as well, as did the other victims. Unable to recognize my dad as my abuser, and therefore my enemy, and not even knowing who I was, I really did "succumb in every battle" like Sun Tzu warns.

It's still hard for me to say my dad is my enemy. I know some people could analyze this to death, but I have trouble saying it because I also know my dad is human. He is just a hurting person. If I really think about it, it's my dad's actions that are the enemy. It just becomes hard to separate his actions from who he is.

A big piece of advice I can give you about moving forward is to first recognize who you are. I had to learn who I was, at my very core, before I could go out into the world and rock it. I'm not saying you have to go to India (although maybe you do) and find yourself. However you go about it, you have to be rooted in the truths about what makes you *you*, otherwise you could get swept up by a gust of wind. Sometimes it's hard to know who you truly are. Maybe you've suffered abuse too, and it's caused you to forget a part of yourself. Or maybe uncovering parts of yourself is scary because you don't know what you might find. I can tell you for sure that there are traits we all have that we wish we didn't. But don't let any of these things keep you from knowing who you are and being proud of that. Like Dr. Seuss said, "Today you are you! That is truer than true! There is no one alive who is you-er than you!" Take time to remember who you are.

But the second part is just as important. You must know who the enemy is as well. If you don't know what you're fighting, how are you supposed to fight it? It's like battling in complete darkness. Fear doesn't exist. Fear of the unknown does. The enemy is the thing that is holding you back. It can be an abusive person, a trauma from your childhood or after, and it can even be that voice in your head that tells you you're not good enough. You've got to fight off all of those things. All those guys are nasty!

Once I knew that it was my dad's abuse that was tormenting me, I could deal with it head-on. I'm not going to lie—it wasn't easy. On the show, I went to a counselor once a week and worked hard to deal with everything. It was hard. Give me a workout, and I'll crush it. Give me a diet plan, and I'll follow it. But the most difficult thing is the mind stuff. The emotional stuff. But if I can do it, you can do it too.

I LIKE TO SAY TO MYSELF

Know your enemy. Know yourself.
Go out and slay.

Chapter 41

Setbacks, Not Steps Back

I was pumped from day one! So when I flew to Colorado for that intensive boot camp, I was ready to go. This is probably tooting my own horn, but I completely crushed boot camp. I lost 121 pounds in three months. You give me a challenge, and I will rise to conquer it. That's just how I am. I set records during that time. My 121 pounds was the most weight any contestant has lost on the show to date. I felt so good.

The process of the show is a year long. After Phase 1, the time at boot camp, all of the contestants go back to their homes for Phase 2 to continue losing weight, using all the helpful tools they acquired over the last three months. It's an exciting time, but it's scary. How would it feel to be home, without Chris or Heidi, without the other contestants who had become my friends, without Dr. Holly, the producers, trainers, dieticians, experts, and everything in between? Honestly, I didn't really think about it.

I traveled home, got on the scale... and wanted to die. I had gained. Words can't describe how awful I felt. I had failed. And you know how much weight I gained? How many pounds caused me to have a complete breakdown? It was two pounds. Two pounds sent me into a downward spiral. I know that seems silly, but I also know you can relate. It wasn't about the number; it was what it meant to gain at all. I was devastated. I took one of those emotional sick days I talked about.

The thing I love most about the show is that everyone involved genuinely cares about you. They want you to succeed for yourself. Yeah, they are making television out of your story, but these people, at their core, just want to get you healthy, emotionally and physically. Which is why when I gained those two pounds, I didn't hesitate to call Chris and Heidi Powell and another producer named Jason. They were there for me like they always have been. They talked me down, saying things I'll never forget (they are a treasure trove of advice and motivation). Chris said, "You know what? You're human. You're upset and rightly so. But it's how you respond right now that will decide whether you have integrity or not. You can be upset, but you don't have to stay in it forever."

He was right, guys. The more I thought about it, the more I realized that all my fears were illogical. I was going to let two pounds upset me? Two pounds?! Heck no! When I was able to take the fear out of it, I could look at the situation rationally. The scale might have read an extra two pounds for any number of reasons. I had just traveled. When you travel, you retain sodium and fluids. I was on a different scale. I was tired. Who knows the real cause? That was irrelevant. I wasn't making excuses, but rationalizing it made it easier for me to overcome.

I decided to live up to the promises I made to the show. I decided to take Chris's advice and have integrity. So the next day, I woke up and crushed it at my workout. Morning after morning, I went even harder than before. I did this for a week before I weighed myself again. It was nerve-wracking. I stepped on that scale and held my breath. You know what happened after I had put in all that hard work? I lost eight pounds. Did you think I was going to say I gained again? Absolutely not. Hard work pays off!

You're going to have setbacks. But if you have enough tools in your tool belt then there is nothing you can't face. You know when you go to an auto repair shop and they always seem to have that little thing to fix your car? They look at the problem and say, "I have just the thing," and then they rummage in the back and produce the thing and the tool to fix it? That's what it's like when you study and acquire skills to grow and heal and, ultimately, lose weight. You would never go into a battle without a weapon. You would never run onto the football field without the proper gear. So please, don't attempt to change your life without the tools that will help you succeed.

You need those things because you are going to fail. Let me say this, I have gained weight other times since my two-pound nightmare. It usually happens when I travel and my body seems to forget everything. But I've also gained because I'm too comfortable. It's so easy to slip back into old routines. Those are failures to me. I can't stand it when I am not at the weight I know I'm capable of maintaining. I may gain a few pounds here or there, but I never go off the deep end. Why? Because I have all this new knowledge—tips and tricks to help get me through those setbacks. Always get back to the things you've learned. You spent the time learning them, might as well use them!

I LIKE TO SAY TO MYSELF

It's just a bump in the road!

Chapter 42

Tommy

While Bruce may have been away from Colorado and all the support he had there during Phase 1, the show wasn't about to leave him feeling alone in Utah during Phase 2. They knew he needed someone to help him feel motivated and teach him while he was back home. Who better than Tommy Hackenbruck, founder of Ute CrossFit?

In the world of CrossFit and fitness, Tommy has become a legend. Competing at the CrossFit Games four times as an individual and three times on the Ute team has solidified Tommy's place with the greats. "Ute has been known for our success at the CrossFit Games… We were the first gym to win back-to-back affiliate cup championships." However, the loving husband and dedicated father of four doesn't let his accomplishments go to his head. And he stresses the impact that Bruce made on his own training and life.

Bruce was fresh off of his high from Phase 1, but his concussion was going to be a major concern at the start of Phase 2. "Chris and Heidi sat down with me and gave me strict instructions. Heidi was adamant about how to deal with Bruce's concussion… Within two sessions of working with

Bruce, I understood why Heidi was like that." Tommy describes a very stubborn man who wanted to work out and crush, no matter the potential brain damage. Bruce was extremely motivated and wanted to reach his goal. At Tommy's gym, they are big on helping individual members reach goals and meeting them where they are. Tommy relied on that when he first started training Bruce, always working around the concussion. "Our first meeting, Bruce was impressed that I was a CrossFit Games guy. That was how I got him to back off [of high intensity]. Because, for the first two weeks, I told him how important it was to do a lot of gymnastics work. I started teaching him a muscle up." And that's when Tommy was floored by Bruce.

A muscle up is an advanced gymnastics movement where you start hanging from a set of rings and pull yourself up until your arms are at your sides and you are supporting your bodyweight on top of the rings. If you've watched Olympic gymnastics, you have seen men do this on the rings. It takes almost inhuman strength and athleticism to accomplish the maneuver. Tommy says, "It's a movement in CrossFit that everyone wants to do. Many people that are in shape can take years to get there." But Bruce learned and achieved a muscle up in a matter of months. And that was before he had even lost all the weight!

Bruce's muscle up left a lasting impression on Tommy. It proved to him that Bruce does something that is crucial to success in life and in weight loss: "He sets ridiculous goals and works toward them, as if he was going to achieve them." But Tommy adds that the craziest part of all about Bruce's high goals is that often he *does* achieve them. Tommy sees a lot of people in their weight-loss journey who reach their goal and then stop. "These people relapse because they are like, 'Yeah, I made it.'" Bruce is the opposite. After he reaches a goal, he sets another. "He doesn't just want to lose weight, he wants to be fit. He doesn't just want to be fit, he wants to be one of the fittest guys in the world... He's continued to set lofty goals."

While Tommy may have helped Bruce along his journey, he reflects on how much Bruce was actually the teacher: "[The year I worked with Bruce] was my best year competing in CrossFit. I was thirty-two, one of the oldest guys there. But I took sixth in the world." Tommy attributes some of that to Bruce. "Bruce was my training partner. We did cardio together. I trained him and coached him, but we would work together a lot too. He inspired me. His passion and relentlessness are contagious." Bruce's inspiration didn't just affect Tommy, it motivated the members of Tommy's gym as well. "He's come in town and coached at my gym. He has an amazing talent for that stuff. I don't even think he realizes how talented he is. He touched a lot of people in my circle."

Bruce also taught Tommy how to help a wider range of people. "We've always wanted to make the gym welcoming and inviting to anyone. We get lots of fit people walking through the door. Bruce inspired and empowered me to meet the other side of the population more. Puts me out of my comfort zone, but it's super rewarding."

Even after Phase 2 and the end of the show, Bruce and Tommy are good friends. "Being able to be part of his life was an honor for me. I don't feel like I did that much for him, but he has done a ton for me."

Chapter 43

Life Is a Season

I know I've talked a lot about the struggles in life. There will be times in your life—many times—when the trials feel overwhelming. Those are dark seasons. The simple truth is that you will go through them and you will survive, hopefully having learned from them on your journey forward. Those are winter months. But spring is coming, I promise. Good, then bad, the cycle will continue. All that means is that you will always go through cold months, but you will also experience many spring times.

There will be seasons in your life when you can't imagine how life could get any better. The show was one of those seasons for me. I met Chris and Heidi, I was losing weight, making friends, lovin' life. When I went back home, who should surprise me but Chris. I loved the week he was with me in Utah. It's amazing how one person can brighten your entire outlook. That was enough for me. But then, one day at one of my football practices, I saw Raghib Ismail, "The Rocket," stepping onto the field. Ismail was a wide receiver for the Oakland Raiders (Raider Nation, baby!). I ran up and we chest bumped. Who gets to say they chest bumped with The

Rocket? He was an awesome guy. We instantly connected. I found out that he had suffered sexual abuse in his past as well. He told me a truth I will never forget, "One of the things you have to learn how to do, as a man, is learn how to overcome." It was great to see how amped he was on life. If he can do it, I can do it. And if I can do it, anyone can do it.

Meeting Raghib Ismail was a huge high in my life. I couldn't believe I got to meet a Raider face-to-face like that. But then Ismail had a little surprise for me. He pulled out four tickets to a Raider's game in Oakland!

So I went down to the Raiders' turf with my mom, my brother, and Chris. We decided to do my six month weigh-in in the tailgate parking lot of the stadium. Doing my weigh-in in front of Raider Stadium was the best ever. I was already about as fired up as you could be. Raider Nation is the best thing my eyes had ever seen. I stood on the scale. My goal was to lose 40 pounds. I lost 47 pounds! That was a total loss of 44 percent of my original body weight. It was a record!

I'm not exaggerating when I say that it was surprise after surprise. The whole thing kept getting better and better. After the weigh-in, Chris took me into the Oakland Coliseum. It was empty, and I got to just bask in it. The sheer magnitude of it was overwhelming. To many, Raider Stadium is considered a dump, in need of some extreme TLC. I don't know how they say that because, to me, it is the most beautiful stadium my eyes have ever seen. I swear I could hear echoes of all of the cheering fans and the games won and lost there. It was a magical moment. After that, we watched the game. It was incredible. I thought that was the end of my trip, and I was 100 percent satisfied. Actually, I was deliriously happy!

The next morning Chris said he had one more surprise for me. He took me to the Raiders' headquarters. Holy heck! We were greeted out front by two rows of cheerleaders. Inside, I got to see the locker room. THE locker room! It was a dream come true. As I was wandering around, looking at the names of all the greats above the lockers, I saw one that read, "PITCHER." I thought, "That's funny. That's my name." That's when they told me they made a special locker for me. I burst into tears. Tears of joy. Up to that point, I had never felt so overwhelmed with joy as I did when I saw that locker.

There are moments in life when you think things can't get any better, but they do. Going to the game, seeing the coliseum, and finding my own locker was like that for me. However, the surprise still wasn't done yet. We went out to the practice field. Even though Chris had said many times that he had one last surprise, he saved the best for last. Chris said, "I want you to meet one of the greatest players of all time." My heart was pounding, my hands got sweaty, and I instantly knew who he was talking about. The one. The only. JERRY RICE! When Jerry walked out onto the field, I felt a kind of happy I've never felt in my life. I said to Chris, "Can I run to him? Can we run?" When Chris gave me the go ahead, I took off toward the legend. We spent the rest of the time running some drills, throwing the ball, and just having fun. The smile on my face was huge, and I kept feeling like, "Dude, is this real? Someone pinch me right now!"

My life had just been completed. It was a milestone, and it was perfect. Never in a million years did I think that would happen to me. The whole experience meant so much to me because football means so much to me. The sport of football saved my life. I wouldn't be the person I am today without it.

That whole story is to emphasize that sometimes life really does get better. There are moments when we receive beyond what we ask or imagine. Those moments will almost always catch us by surprise. Always remember there are seasons of spring. It doesn't mean there won't be bad seasons. If you're going through a rough time right now, remember: Spring is coming.

I LIKE TO SAY TO MYSELF

It's only a season.

Chapter 44

Don't Be a Dude

Y ou know how some guys have this weird problem with asking for directions? If you're a dude, you know you've done it. I've done it. I'll admit it. And I get lost on the road because of it sometimes.

Well, I think it's the same thing for people when they need to ask for help. It's hard to ask for help. I know that it makes me feel embarrassed. I feel like I'm bothering the person I'm asking. But mainly I feel like I've failed. If I need to go to someone to help me, then that means I'm not strong enough to help myself. For a long time, that made me feel weak. But it's so not true! There is absolutely no shame in reaching out. I've already told you how I learned the very, very hard way that it didn't help me at all to try and get through something so difficult by myself.

The show really taught me the value in reaching out and asking for a lifeline. The producers, counselors, trainers, other contestants, and especially Chris and Heidi were big on telling me to call them whenever, for whatever.

When I was back home in Utah, in Phase 2 of my transformation, I had a lot of great things happen to me. Tommy was great. Chris's visit was great. Seeing the Raiders was heaven. But I was struggling. I had learned all this great, new stuff, like how to handle things mentally, how to eat, and how to work out, but I was having trouble applying these new techniques to an old lifestyle. It was so easy to fall back into what I had been doing for all of those years. At least this time I had the clarity to see immediately that this was not going to work. I called up Chris and Heidi and just said, "You know what? It's not working here." They didn't shame me, they only encouraged me. I told them I needed help, and they said, "We have just the thing."

There were a few seasons of the show before mine, so it wasn't their first rodeo. They knew contestants might struggle to apply what they had learned in Colorado. True and lasting transformation doesn't happen in a day. It takes hours, days, months, and even years to truly learn to use all of the tools and to be able to move forward. So the show had a house set up in Arizona (where Chris and Heidi live) where contestants could stay for as long as they needed to. I raised my white flag and asked for help, so they let me live there.

I'm so glad. Some of my friends from the show were there, as well as other contestants. Everyone was in the same boat, and we were all working together. During this process, you're going to have to recondition your brain. It's like learning to walk all over again, but it's all mental. That takes a lot of dedication and application. It was much easier to put to use all of the tools I got in Phase 1 when I was around people who were there to help. It helped me feel like I was being held accountable. During Phase 2, after asking for help, I ended up crushing it again and lost 47 pounds. I had now lost over 40 percent of my original body weight. And more importantly, I had met my goal for Phase 2.

Today, all that practice has made the techniques habits. I still have to work hard, but it's different. I am able to hold myself accountable. I'm not saying I don't have those days when I struggle. But now I'm quick to ask for help. If you don't ask for directions, you'll probably get lost. If you don't ask for help, it's the same.

I LIKE TO SAY TO MYSELF

Just ask for help!

Chapter 45

No Rope

When I was living in Arizona, the weight continued to melt off. I was still crushing it. I was living in a house with my friends. Chris and Heidi were close by. I was loving it. If you've been on a weight-loss journey, I'm sure you can relate to what happened next.

When you're losing weight and cruising along, you gain confidence, which is good. But sometimes too much confidence can lead to feeling comfortable. I'm not saying you should feel uncomfortable all of the time, but being too cozy can cause you to slack off. It's like a warm bed in the morning. It's comfortable, but you can't sleep in it all day. Enjoy it when you should, but eventually you have to throw the covers off and let the freezing morning air jar you awake!

I can tell you that I was for sure feeling great at my weigh-in on one particular Sunday. I stepped on that scale, and sure enough, I had lost weight. I felt good and ate my reset meal without any guilt or fear. I deserved it. We all deserve a reset meal. They help. They work. But then something weird happened. Early in the week, I started thinking about maybe having a little candy bar. I thought I was doing good, so I deserved that too. I also thought it would be okay since I was losing so consistently, and I was keeping up with all the other stuff. I thought it wasn't going to hurt anybody. So I had a candy bar. No big deal. At the end of the week, I stepped on the scale, and BOOM, I had lost weight again. So now I was thinking that candy bar wasn't such a bad idea. It didn't affect me at all. I was stoked that I could have a little treat now and then. I had completely forgotten that that was exactly what my reset meal was for. The reset meal is the treat. But yeah, I forgot.

And so the slippery slope began. I thought that if I could have one candy bar, maybe I could have two candy bars. So I had two candy bars the next week. I went to my weigh-in on Sunday, and BOOM, I had lost weight again. As I was going on in this process, I went from one candy bar a week, to two, to three, to four candy bars a week! I was continuing to lose weight. I was doing really well. Life was good.

Fast forward to a week and a half before they were going to film the finale. This was almost the end. I had my skin surgery and recovered. I had already lost 50 percent of my body weight. I was feeling pumped. As I was going along that week, I was feeling more and more comfortable. I was eating a little extra protein here and a few extra carbs there. Some little treats here and there. But I was confident that I would crush it.

I didn't have a scale in the house. I don't like them. I hate weighing myself during the week because it screws up my mental game. Three days before the filming of the finale, Heidi stopped by to see how we were all doing. She had a scale with her. I got on the scale and thought nothing of it. I got off and asked Heidi, "Will I be okay?" Heidi said, "Well, you'll be fine." Except, here's the thing: I know Heidi really well and I can read her really well, and the way she said it wasn't good. Nobody likes giving bad news, especially Heidi. All she wants is to encourage people. The tone in her voice and the look on her face said it all, though. She didn't tell me how much I weighed. Later that night, I thought I would figure out for myself what happened. I found a scale somewhere and weighed myself. I had been around 186 to 187 pounds. BAM, I was 207 pounds! I went into a deep panic really quickly. I thought I had completely failed. I wasn't at the end of my rope because there was no rope to even hang on to. It was over for me in that moment. I was done. I packed my bags. I was going to quit. I texted Heidi and told her it was over, then I stormed out of the house. It was late at night, and I just walked the streets.

The next morning, I was ready to quit. I had thrown in the towel because I was so upset. I wasn't even going to be 50 percent for the finale weigh-in. I was going to show that I gained weight. It was going to be so depressing. Here I am, the guy everyone thought was crushing it, the guy everyone thought was so positive this whole time. It would ruin my episode. I had the worst thoughts swimming around in my head.

However, Chris and Heidi weren't going to let me go that easily. They weren't going to give up on me or let me give up on myself. Heidi came and picked me up and took me to their house. I told them I felt like a failure. I had gone 362 days being pretty dang solid. Yeah, I had my mess-ups here and there, but nothing that bad. And now, three days before my finale, I screwed it all up, right before the finish line. That was eating at me so much because it didn't show my integrity. Everything I said I would do, it all would go down the drain. Then Chris started building me up. He and Heidi reminded me of all the truths I had forgotten. They showed me how far I had come and helped me believe in myself again. They brought me back to integrity and pumped me up. I had acquired all of the tools. I had put in all of the work. Now I just had to do it a little bit longer.

I didn't go home. I didn't quit. The next three days I put in a lot of hard work. I was still nervous, but I had to set that aside and focus on the task in front of me. I couldn't think about what would happen if I didn't reach my goal. I couldn't think about people thinking I was a fraud. All I could do was what I could do.

The day of the finale came, and I was nervous but excited as all get out. I stood on that scale and the number was in. 181 pounds. I had reached my goal.

The moral of the story is this: Everything won't always be hunky-dory. Even three days before the finale—the final weigh-in—I wanted to quit the show, and I thought I had failed. What I'm saying is that you're never done with this process. You're going to be defeated and you will feel like you let yourself down. It's not necessarily a bad thing because your integrity is what's most important to you. I think that's what hit me hard. Because I said I was going to do it. And I fulfilled it all the way to the very end. It was one of the biggest blessings in disguise. It was one of the most eye-opening experiences to realize that you can't ever figure it all out. It's impossible. We are always growing. So I'm grateful for that experience. All smiles and everything. It's still a grind, every single day.

I LIKE TO SAY TO MYSELF

It's a brand-new life, Bruce. Live it.

Chapter 46

Bob

"I actually didn't like him when I first met him. We were both offensive linemen and coaches as well, so I thought we would have a lot in common. But Bruce was standoffish when I met him," Bob Brenner says. Bob was on season three of *Extreme Weight Loss*, the one right before Bruce's. He was brought in to help the new contestants for season four and met Bruce at the facility in Colorado. What Bob didn't know at the time was that he met Bruce during his severe concussion. Later, their paths crossed again and his feelings completely changed. They were assigned to be motivational coaches together and that really solidified their friendship. Their love of working out and sports connected them, but their shared experience on the show bonded them. To be part of a show like *Extreme Weight Loss* is like being a part of a very small fraternity.

Bob was a detective in the narcotics department of the local police department in Wisconsin for twenty-three years. He loved his job and still loves his life. This family man radiates kindness, a quality that is simple, yet so rare. He has seen it all and still manages to be warm, friendly, and connect with people on a level that makes them feel like he truly cares. He is thankful for his life: weight gain, weight loss, and all. All he wants is to use his story to help others. He's created a program called Real Transformation to do just that. He is also an author (*Live an Extreme Life: Losing the Weight and Gaining My Purpose*), a motivational speaker, and a life coach.

His grateful, love-of-life outlook is similar to Bruce's and one of the reasons they have remained such close friends. Bob was able to help Bruce through the transition off the show. He told Bruce, "When you get into maintaining, it's going to suck, so call me." Bruce did call him and now they build each other up. "He and I have gotten a little out of control on an indulgence meal. When I need to go through a confession, I'll talk to Bruce about how I have to be on track. There's no judgment from Bruce."

Bob and Bruce have become very involved in a transformation program. It's a twelve-week program to help kickstart a lifelong transformation. They share a similar dream about helping others. "We both made a conscious decision that we wanted to help people moving forward. We wanted to help people that had our struggles. In order for us to be authentic, we have to live the lifestyle," Bob explains. The program not only helps the people participating, it helps Bob and Bruce be held accountable too, which is a big part of maintaining a new lifestyle.

One of Bob's favorite stories about Bruce involves Bruce's classic forgetfulness. Bob and Bruce were in town for a transformation and decided to get a workout in. Bob is more into cardio and Bruce is more into CrossFit, so they went their separate ways, knowing they had to be back by a certain time. "I told him to bring a towel, but Bruce would forget his hand if it wasn't attached," Bob says, and true to form, Bruce had forgotten a towel. He needed to shower, and there was a strict time frame, so he just ran and found a towel in the lost and found. When they met up, Bob asked how Bruce showered without a towel: "He said, 'I don't know, I just kind of grabbed a towel.'" The story stands out to both men because they found a deeper truth in it. "Sometimes in life, you just find a towel and you just go," Bob explains. You can anticipate and prepare, but there will be moments when you need to adapt and adjust spontaneously. It's part of life.

For Bob, Bruce's appeal is simple. "He was just a guy that had been through hell. For him to have the attitude and be the guy he is, just inspired me. When I hear the phrase, 'when God made that person, he broke the mold,' I think of Bruce. That guy walks to the beat of his own drum. His humor is spontaneous; it comes out of left field. He loves life and he's fun to be around, forgetful and all."

Chapter 47

The Cookie Aisle

When I was a big guy, I shared a lot of things. People are always giving me tickets to a game or an event, and I would share them. I happily shared my energy and my time. But there was one thing I didn't share and that was my food. I was the guy who would order an appetizer that was *only* for me. I look back and think, how ridiculous! I wasn't even aware I had this weird food-hoarding behavior at the time. I only learned it later when my friends told me. I'm not that guy anymore. That's because I usually don't even order an appetizer anymore (unless it's my reset meal). It was one of a million sacrifices I've made. Sacrifice is a big part of a weight-loss journey. It's stupid hard. The cravings are crazy. But let me tell you something that makes it easier: Stop thinking of it as giving up something and start thinking about it as making a payment toward a new you.

I had to give up so much the year I was on the show. Not just food, but I gave up my life in Utah for a while. I gave up my friends. I gave up most of my free time. But it didn't feel that bad because I knew I was working toward something. I had a goal in the end.

When I got home, the transition was rough. There were lots of distractions. All of my favorite go-to restaurants were still there. And the cookie aisle... don't even get me started. It's super hard not to just take a little cruise down the row of treats. Some strategies really do help, like avoiding the grocery store when you're hungry. Obviously, that doesn't always work. Sometimes when I'm driving home from dinner or a good workout, my mind goes to the Reese's Pieces at the gas station right on my route. I try to convince myself that a little bit of candy won't hurt. Or the biggest excuse: that I deserve it. But then I hear another voice in my head. The one that reminds me of what my goals are. It reminds me how far I've come. It reminds me of all the good things about making sacrifices. That positive voice becomes louder than the negative one. It took me a long time to develop that. It's going to take you a while too, but you're on the right track, right now, reading this very sentence.

I'm going to be really honest, trying to rid yourself of mental and physical baggage is the hardest thing ever. It involves a huge amount of sacrifice. You have to lose to gain. Physical changes without mental changes are only short term. But once you understand at your core why you're doing it, once you have integrity, you will be able to walk by the cookies without even looking.

Why? Because every time you make a sacrifice, that's a payment toward an investment in you. You're giving up junk food so that you can gain a healthier life. Every time you put down the double cheeseburger, that's a payment. When a donut is sounding really good, but you don't eat it, that's one more contribution to the piggy bank that is yourself. The cravings will fade, but they will never go away entirely.

However, with each craving, you have a choice about how to "spend" it. Are you going to eat it up? Or invest it?

This idea isn't just about food; it applies to actual money as well. You think you can't afford a gym membership? Think about how much money you spend on eating out every day. Yeah, you might be eating cheap fast food, like I used to, but it adds up quickly when you have to buy enough to fuel a morbidly obese body. It's not like you're ordering one thing from the dollar menu. I used to spend at least fifteen to twenty dollars at Taco Bell. You know just as well as I do that that is way too many tacos. Cut back five dollars a day, and you could have an awesome gym membership. You might think you're strong enough to work out at home. Maybe you are part of a minuscule group of people who can be that self-motivated, but if you're like me (or anyone else), I can tell you that being a part of a gym helps for sure. Spend the money. Invest in yourself. It's the best decision you could possibly make. A good way to ensure that your investment is protected is to have accountability. Having another person, or multiple people, to hold you accountable is like having insurance. When you spend the money to get a gym membership, take advantage of the opportunity to work out with someone. It will make it more likely that you won't quit. It's a way to get your return on your investment.

If anyone knows about being broke, it's me. I've had financial struggles for as long as I can remember. But where there's a will, there's a way. I believe that.

When you make payments to yourself, both mentally and monetarily, just like any good investment, it will come back to you with interest. You will be surprised at how all the little sacrifices—the little payments—add up. And an even cooler thing that happens is that after a while you'll feel the sacrifices less and less and the gains more and more. There's no feeling quite as good as that.

I LIKE TO SAY TO MYSELF

With each sacrifice, you're making
payments toward your future.

Chapter 48

Integrity

I never knew how long the audition process was on a show like *Extreme Weight Loss*. It's crazy. I understand it's important, but there is a lot of stuff and you begin to feel like it won't end. One day, Chris and Heidi surprised us at casting finals. I'll never forget it. Chris said something that really registered with me. It's something I remember to this day.

He looked at all of us and said, "The number one thing that none of you have is integrity." It sounds shocking, but something even more shocking is that his comment had little to no effect on me at first. In fact, it didn't really hurt at all. Chris went on, "None of you are keeping your promises." The more he expanded on it, the more I was like, "Now, hang on, Chris..." However, after he began talking about having integrity and keeping promises, I realized he was right. I wasn't living up to the best me. I wasn't keeping my word. Chris explained that if you say you're going to run 20 minutes on the treadmill, you can't stop at 19:59.

That's what integrity looks like. Do the 20 minutes. Do not stop an inch before the finish line! Go all the way through. That's what champions do because champions have integrity. Even if no one else sees, you must do it for you.

Even now, to this day, when I'm on the treadmill and I start looking around and I think no one's there, I think, "Do I finish my workout?" I can hear Chris's voice, "Don't stop at 19:59!" When I'm as tired as can be, when I don't want to complete a workout—or fulfill a commitment—that story comes into my head. When he made that such a big deal. That's how much of an impact it had.

Integrity is about keeping promises, but it's also about making promises too. It's important to set goals for yourself and tell people what those goals are. It's also important to make realistic promises to yourself so that you can fulfill them. After the show, I struggled. Keeping your integrity is a 24/7 commitment. There are no breaks from integrity. You have to devote yourself to being the best you can be. You have to go the full 20 minutes.

When the show was over, all of the cameras were gone, and I was home—that's when the thoughts started creeping back in. The negative thoughts. I also got comfortable. I gained a little bit of weight during that time, nothing crazy. Everyone kept telling me I was fine and that I looked great. But deep down I knew I wasn't maintaining my integrity and living up to the promises I made to myself. I had all the tools, and I wasn't using them to the best of my ability. You know why? Pride. The thing that holds us back from having integrity is pride. I was worried about telling people I was falling behind a little. I was worried about sharing a new goal because I didn't want people to know. I made up all this pressure from the other contestants. They all looked up to me, and I didn't want to let them down. But more importantly, I didn't want to look bad. It was my ego. I couldn't show them I had weaknesses. They would always say, "Look, Bruce is killing it." I didn't want to let them know I was struggling.

But that's ridiculous! Enough is enough. It wasn't always hunky-dory, but I was going to swallow my pride and have integrity again. It was time for me to put up or shut up. I decided to sign up for a physique show. Not only that, but I posted a video about it. Now everyone would know. But I like that. I like being held accountable.

As soon as I decided to do the physique show, I started battling against myself. I remember I was driving home and I really wanted some Reese's Pieces, and I thought, "I could start tomorrow." It was crazy! Everything I've been blessed with, all the opportunities I've had, all the people in my life who care, and I'm going to throw it away on candy? Why would I do that? Heck no, gosh dang it! I'm not going to do that. I had to come back to integrity.

Integrity also means practicing gratitude. I talked myself down on that drive home by appreciating everything in my life. I decided that if I stopped for a treat, if I was breaking the promises I made to myself, I wouldn't be acting like a good person.

I made it home without stopping. It was a little victory. But it's those little victories that add up and lead to big change, which leads to being truly happy.

When you're able to mentally and emotionally overcome something, that brings a kind of happiness that no amount of money or any thing can give you. Nothing can bring you the happiness you feel when you have personal fulfillment, not anything... except maybe the Raiders winning the Super Bowl. I'm just kidding!... (I'm really not).

I LIKE TO SAY TO MYSELF

You have integrity.

Chapter 49

Ignite the Day

When the idea of integrity finally clicked for me, I realized that there were things I was already doing with integrity. That's one thing that has been encouraging to me along this journey: I wasn't always failing at everything. Sure, I've had to learn a lot. I've had to recondition my brain and thought process. I've been disciplined, and I've taken to heart all the things that Chris and Heidi have said about integrity. There have been moments in this process where I thought I was just a failure. But what I see now is that, while there were some definite black marks, I have some inherent good within me too. No one is all good or all bad—all failure or all success. The more I learned about integrity, the more I could see how I actually had some of those traits already. For instance: I have always liked to ignite the day. Even when I was 400 pounds. That's why I did naked squats and got pumped every morning. But there was another way I was exercising integrity and igniting the day without even realizing it.

Here it is: I always like to say a positive thing to three people before 10 a.m. Even better if it's a stranger. I know it

183

sounds simple, but something so easy could mean the world to someone else. It's a way to spread joy and life to those around you.

My dad would always tear me down. He did it so that he could manipulate me. I've heard that when your parent demonstrates a trait you don't like, you either act exactly like them or do the opposite. Luckily, in this case, I did the opposite. I never want anyone to feel like they aren't good enough. I never felt good enough. I was always desperate for acceptance and love and look where it got me. But now that I understand that I am loved, I feel like I can go out and fly! I want everyone I meet to feel that way too. I recommend waking up in the morning, ready to ignite the day, and seeing what happens when you say a positive thing to three people before 10 a.m.

When I get around people, I can't help but notice the positives about them. I'm not trying to toot my own horn. It's just the reality of who I am. I'm lucky in that way. When you say something positive to someone you don't know, sometimes it opens up a conversation. And that conversation may lead to a friendship and that friendship may change your life.

Because I was on the show, it allowed me to take my igniting-the-day technique to so many places in my life I never thought I would go. The show brought me into a whole other world, filled with new and inspiring people. Because I've lost the weight, I have met people I never in a million years would've known, let alone been good friends with. I'm now friends with world class athletes, TV personalities, and people changing the world, not to mention Chris and Heidi Powell, my second family. I began the show with my family and an absolutely killer set of friends and coaches. I never thought my life could get any more full when it came to who

I had in it. But how much my world has expanded since the show, and the people I've come in contact with, is staggering and incredible.

Now, when I wake up and ignite the day, I'm able to say positive things to complete strangers during my speaking events. I am so thankful for the strangers that approach me after an event and tell me their stories about how they have overcome trials in their own lives. They inspire me.

So get out there and seize the day! Get pumped! And show some love!

I LIKE TO SAY TO MYSELF

Say something positive to three people before 10 a.m.

Chapter 50

Mike and Jake

"I have a guy you have to meet. He lost 200 pounds. He's incredible." That was the text that Mike Cazayoux received from one of his close friends. This was back in 2014 when Mike, two-time CrossFit Games team champion and exercise specialist, was about to launch the podcast for his company, Brute Strength Training. Mike agreed to interview Bruce. So he hopped in the car with Jake Hutton, one of his coaches and contributors to Brute Strength, and they drove from Salt Lake City to Colorado to meet Bruce and interview him for the podcast.

Mike is no stranger to overcoming struggles of his own. "I was an all-American child," Mike says. His father was a congressman and state representative and his mother was loving and nurturing at home. Still, Mike says he was destined to get in trouble because of the boredom he felt in a small town. Long story short, Mike got in with the wrong crowd, which led him down a dark path, ending with a crack and heroin addiction. Rehab, AA, and therapy eventually worked for Mike and he's been sober ever since (eight years and counting). He's married to Adee (founder of Working Against Gravity, a company dedicated to helping people have a healthy relationship with food). But it was during that tumultuous time that Mike acquired the tools he would use in his own business, Brute Strength Training. And it was how he would later relate to Bruce.

Jake is married and a father of three. He's also a big name in the athletic—specifically CrossFit—world. A two-time CrossFit Games competitor, Jake is now using his own training techniques to help others. He does online programming for people all over the world who are looking for a healthier lifestyle. He has worked alongside Mike and also Steve Cook, a huge name in the fitness realm.

On their way from Utah, Jake drove and, as Mike describes, "I watched Bruce's episode in the car on our way to Colorado and I was floored. It's such a heart-wrenching story. Seeing the positive person he is, after having gone through all of that, is incredible." After seeing such fanfare surrounding Bruce, Mike was expecting a lot. "I had high expectations. After meeting Bruce, he met them and more. This guy goes hard."

Jake had a similar first impression when he met Bruce. "He has tons of energy. But at the same time Bruce can just hang. He fit in with me and my friends immediately." Jake and Mike recognized one of the reasons why Bruce has been so successful when they worked out with him for the first time. Mike, Jake, Bruce, and Caleb, from Project Rise Fitness, decided to create teams and compete against each other. Even though they had just met, when it came time to pair, Jake knew who he wanted as his partner. "I wanted Bruce... the CrossFit workout was full of farmer's carries, sleds, and a lot of things requiring throwing weight around. I figured Bruce had a good engine because he had just been doing long workouts on the show. Plus, doing a 200-pound farmer's carry when you just lost 200 pounds is basically like working out with your old weight." Despite the fact that Mike and Caleb were both seasoned athletes who had competed at the CrossFit Games, Jake and Bruce "smoked them. We crushed." But it wasn't all because he had been working out for the show or that he was lighter. Jake points out another advantage Bruce had: "He has a background in athletics. He has a competitive edge that way. He's one of the most competitive dudes I've ever met."

Even though Jake knows the reason why Bruce gained the weight ("I know it was because of soda!") he also knows the reason why Bruce keeps it off. "Honestly, I think it's because he's always just been super positive. The thing that stands out for me about Bruce, and why so many people love him, is that he's the only person I've ever met that doesn't have ill intentions toward anybody. I think that's why he has such a big touch on those he meets. He sees the best in everyone." Bruce calls Jake almost every day just to say "what's up" and talk about his workouts, all of which are tailored specifically for Bruce by Jake himself. Jake does what he does for all his clients. He creates a unique program for Bruce to help him stay lean and strong. But he also helps him push toward his goals. And he is thankful to know Bruce: "He's one of my best friends now."

Mike has had a similar revelation about Bruce's seemingly unwavering positivity. When it comes to workouts, Mike sees something good in something that could be bad: "He's a little bit reckless. He brings himself to the point of vomiting. He has a higher pain tolerance than most people. He pushes himself to his physical limit. He goes so quickly, tries so hard, that is the reason for his success." Mike says that Bruce has never been concerned what others might think of him when he works out, even when he was 400 pounds. Bruce is an inspiration to Mike in his own training endeavors at Brute Strength. "I like working with the average Joe. I like helping people that can't do a full squat do a full squat. I want to help someone lift a suitcase or some other everyday movement they couldn't do before. The other thing that I love, this goes for coaching anyone... is to see the mental and emotional transformation." And when it comes to Bruce, Mike can't help but see Bruce's own transformation. "Just seeing how someone can go through that much, both personal and interpersonally, and come out as positive and radiant as he is has literally made me a better person. When I want to complain and I'm around Bruce, I have to stop because I think, 'What am I complaining about?' The way he attacks a room and brings light to it is inspiring to me."

Chapter 51

Love Ripples

always felt like my dad and I had the best father-son relationship and that no two people could be closer. But I also constantly felt like I wasn't good enough for my dad. A weird mix. He would tell me all of the time that I needed to be like so-and-so because people liked them. People liked my dad. All his self-worth came from what others thought of him so, naturally, he taught me that as well. It was a lie. But I didn't know that at the time. He was so critical of me and told me so many other lies that I began, from an early age, to think I wasn't worth liking, let alone loving.

I always tried to be everything to everyone because I wanted them to love me. When my dad went to prison, I still didn't have his approval, so I craved it from anyone and everyone. I was a loving friend, but I had crippling insecurities.

I met Skyler just after high school at a flag football game. We were on opposite teams. I'm a passionate guy in general, but especially about sports, so I think I got a little heated... okay, a lot heated. I thought Skyler's team was doing something wrong, so I made him my enemy. I couldn't stand him. I tried to fight him, but Skyler, being so patient and calm, didn't fight back. (Also, I was much bigger than him.) However, things changed when another mutual acquaintance came into the picture. Have you ever heard the phrase, "The enemy of my enemy is my friend"? Skyler and I realized we both had an intense dislike for a certain dude, which brought us together, and we've been friends ever since. We realized how stupid our original fight was and became best buds.

Skyler has always been there for me. There's not a thing the guy hasn't done for me. I know that whatever happens to me in my life, I can call Skyler, any second, any minute of the day, and he'll be there for me. There's something about him that's just awesome. He and his entire family accepted me with open arms. Any time I would be in a bad place, Skyler would be there. He was there when my dad went to the parole hearing. He was the only friend who showed up that day. Skyler was like, "I'll be there." It wasn't even a question, he was just like, "I'll be there." At my six-month milestone, Skyler was like, "I'll be there." At my ninety-day weigh-in... the finale... every time.

He sat right behind me during my dad's parole hearing. You create a special bond with the person who was there on a day like that. It's an experience unlike any other—you can't even describe what it was like.

Skyler saw me at my worst. I was always talking negatively about myself. Then I would feel embarrassed about it, so I would get insecure and the cycle continued. One time I was hanging out at Skyler's house. I invited someone over, and Skyler joked and gave me a hard time for inviting someone to his house. I didn't get that it was a joke and I felt so stupid. I got so upset that I started jabbing my forehead with my keys. Skyler immediately said he was just joking. Then I was embarrassed. Skyler loved me, but I couldn't see it because I didn't love myself. Even though I tried really hard, I didn't think I was good enough.

However, you never know what impact you have on people. When I was on the show, I got help to work through my feelings of inadequacy. I began to learn how to love myself. When you love yourself, a beautiful thing happens—people start loving you even more. I couldn't see my emotional transformation or the light I was casting on others. I still continued to doubt myself. After we finished filming, one single email would change all of that.

Rod was a contestant on the show. People always say that I am larger than life. If that's true, I don't even know what they would say about Rod... larger than the universe? Rod was a high school drama teacher, and on the show, Rod was a party everywhere he went. His natural showmanship meant a good time. His encouragement was infectious. He was just an all-around good dude.

His heart was so big. He was an inspiration to me, which is why when Heidi forwarded me an email Rod sent to the producers, I was floored to learn he felt the same about me. That email was the final piece of the puzzle that helped me believe I was worth something.

Heidi wrote:

> It's important you see this. We want you to see what we see. You are loved, Bruce. SO much. You are here on this earth for a reason.

Here's what Rod had written:

This experience is enriching and transformative in so many ways. You guys all obviously know exactly what you are doing as this group of us... I have never been a part of anything like this. It's like a brotherhood. Or a fellowship. Our connections to each other—most of us, anyway, is so strong. Week two or not, we all get each other and support each other and really do love each other. I think it's chemical—something about the mix, and that includes all of you guys too—Mr. Powell, Mrs. Powell, Ms. Settlemier, Ms. Brothers, Mr. Assmus, and Mr. Roth (whose presence is ALWAYS felt... in a great way, J. D.).

I love all these guys—and some, like Georgeanna, and David, and Brandi, and Jayce are truly my peeps. My new roomie Josh is becoming a close buddy.

But there's something kind of extraordinary about Bruce.

I know J. D. saw it early and all of you have seen it since. All of us KNOW it. That boy is a leader, you guys. A true motivator. A deep soul. He just is—he is more powerful than he knows, which makes him even more dynamic. I watch Bruce at our workouts—I am inspired and moved to do better because he always, always gives his best. And when he finishes his challenges and tasks (usually first), he has the energy and grace to come support the rest of us—sometimes verbally by pumping us up, but mostly he does it in ingenious, quiet ways: running or walking next to you so that you find the stamina you didn't know you still possessed to finish and go stronger; listening to you while you share your feelings and giving expert advice or just encouragement. Sometimes his smile and laugh can just bring you into a good place.

I should probably send this to him... maybe I will, but every day you guys... EVERY SINGLE DAY this man does something that lifts my soul a little bit. A little higher.

He is for me what I know I am for thousands of students. He is my teacher. Soon he will be one for the world. I plan to know him and to be friends with him the rest of my life. That's the thing about Bruce. He's the real deal. And I am lucky I made a soul connection with him.

So thanks, you guys, for bringing this amazing, astonishing, astounding (all the "A's") man into my world. Into OUR world.

I think we are all the better for knowing him. Don't you?

Love, Rod

Rod said he planned to be friends with me the rest of his life. Sadly, that would be true. I have trouble talking about this, but his hard and fast life caught up with him after the show. He ended up going into a diabetic shock and dying. I was devastated. I still am.

His letter brings tears to my eyes. I'm humbled and inspired by his words. Sometimes you don't realize the impact you're making on other people. I started loving myself on the show, and in turn, I was able to love others. What my dad said about me wasn't true. Rod's letter helps me remember that, and so do all of my castmates. I wouldn't be here today without them. They have changed my life in so many ways.

I LIKE TO SAY TO MYSELF

You are making a positive impact on those around you.

Chapter 52

Alexa

"Whatever girl ends up with him will be really lucky." That was Alexa's first thought after seeing Bruce Pitcher. However, the way they crossed paths is not what you would expect.

Some may describe her as shy, but Alexa is just an incredibly relaxed individual who is confident enough to feel comfortable being alone. She personifies the expression "still waters run deep" and hardly anything seems to faze her. Her long brown hair flows down to her waist, her almond eyes look at you intently with kindness, and when she smiles, which is often, her subtle dimples make you feel the goodness that radiates from her heart.

Alexa describes herself as being rational and logical. She definitely keeps her cool in almost any situation, which is why when she first saw Bruce she didn't know how to process what she felt.

"I remember so clearly. I don't even know why," Alexa begins the story of how she met Bruce. Her roommate was out and she was at her apartment alone that night. A cozy night in meant relaxing on the couch, browsing the channels. Alexa was looking for something to watch when an episode of *Extreme Weight Loss* caught her eye. She didn't watch the show religiously, but the description intrigued her. The episode was a rerun. And you guessed it, it also happened to be Bruce's episode. "I started watching and I was mesmerized," she says. During the two-hour episode, Alexa describes what she calls a unique experience. "You could see everything about him changing. It was so crazy. This guy was amazing and he's going to have an amazing life. You watch those shows all the time and you feel indifferent, but I felt instantly connected and wanted the best for him. I wanted him to be happy." She was so moved by Bruce's story that that's when she thought to herself, "Whatever girl ends up with him will be really lucky." She couldn't believe that someone could be so forgiving, loving, and caring after living through that nightmare. The episode ended, but Alexa would continue to think about Bruce and pray for only good things to come to him.

Little did she know that, miraculously, only a few days later, good things would come to her.

"My friend and I went to a Rockies game. After, we went to Denver's most popular bar." Alexa and her friend were talking and people watching for "maybe two minutes," when a guy walked by and Alexa did a double take. It was Bruce! "I couldn't believe it." Normally an incredibly reserved person, Alexa could not help herself and decided to go talk to him. She had to let him know what an impact his story had made on her. Bruce was visiting the bar with a bunch of the crew from the show. Since his season had wrapped, Bruce was helping out on the next season. He was standing with a camera guy, a production coordinator—people like that—but close enough in the busy bar that Alexa was able to just walk up to his circle. She asked if he was on the show and the rest is history.

"I'm a really hard person to open up, I don't open up easily. I'm never super romantic in that way like, 'oh my gosh, I like this guy, we are going to be together forever.' With Bruce, I felt something was so different. I was slow to say it. I didn't want to get my hopes up. But that first night we met, I felt so comfortable with him. It felt right."

Alexa's only regret about their unique and romantic meet-cute was that she didn't tell her mom about her feelings before she met Bruce. "I'm so annoyed I didn't tell my mom because now she will never believe that I started to fall in love with Bruce before I ever met him face-to-face."

Chapter 53

My Anchor

From the time that I first met him, all he
really wanted was to find someone. It was
in the deepest part of his heart to get married
and have a family.

             —Bailey Wood

W hen you're 400 pounds, you don't ever imagine that you'll find love. Who was going to love me when I could hardly walk up a flight of stairs without getting out of breath? Who would love me when I looked and felt like a hideous tub of lard? It sounds stupid, but if you've been very overweight, you know you've said things like that to yourself. And most of all, whenever I thought of finding love, I could hear my dad's voice in the back of my mind always telling me I wasn't good enough.

My dad used to tell me he was the only person who really cared about me. When he would be critical of me and put me down, he would tell me it was because he was making me a better person. Looking at it now, I see that I viewed his con-trolling behavior as loving behavior because he said it was

so. I believed him when he said no one would ever love me.
But even though I was never exposed to real love—pure love,
true love—somehow my heart always yearned for it. I craved
something I had never tasted.

It doesn't take very long to see that I'm an emotional guy.
I'm proud to wear my heart on my sleeve. And I'm not embarrassed to say that I'm a romantic at heart. Just because I
thought I never would get married didn't mean I didn't want
to get married. I was more than willing to share my heart
with a wife and children, but I just figured it wasn't in the
cards for me. How quickly life can change...

Shortly after the show, I met her. The girl who would forever be my anchor. The girl who would make me think, every
time I look at her, "I'm the luckiest guy in the world." The
girl who would show me through words and actions what
it meant to be loved by another human being. The girl who
would help erase all of the lies my dad told me about love
and write in the truth.

I met Alexa in Colorado, at a sports bar called ViewHouse.
It was the Fourth of July, three days after my birthday. I didn't
know it at the time, but I had just met the woman who would
be the best gift I would ever receive for all birthdays to come.

I'll never forget our first date. I decided to take her to a
Rockies game. The Rockies were playing the Padres. Obviously, sports are very important to me, so I figured I should
test the waters a bit and see how she would react.

When I went to pick her up, I couldn't figure out where
she lived. I had missed a couple of streets and felt a little
lost. I was stressing a bit because of nerves. Finally, I got to
her apartment. Alexa was waiting outside. I can still see her
standing there, one foot against the wall and the other on
the ground, casually looking down at her phone. Seeing her

waiting there had a calming effect on me that has yet to go away. Normally my love wears flowy dresses, like the angel she is, but for the game she was rocking shorts and a Rockies tank top... a good sign.

We met up with some other *Extreme Weight Loss* buddies and headed to the game. Our seats were pretty dang good: third base side, about fifteen rows up. I took my seat next to Alexa, and within moments, I was floored by this girl.

A little back story: Growing up, my friends always told me I needed to find a girl who loved sports. At that time, finding a girl who would love me seemed like an impossible feat, so I never even considered asking God for a girl who loved sports too. But after two seconds of watching the game with Alexa, I knew that I had been blessed with a girl who knew her stuff.

Alexa impressed me that night. She didn't just know the game. She knew the team stats, the strategy, and even the history. Best of all, she loved it! How could a girl be so smart, so beautiful, and so knowledgeable about sports?! I hit the jackpot. Cha-ching, baby!

The game went on, and we were all feeling a little hungry. As we were searching for the perfect game-day meal, I started to worry. How was I supposed to explain to Alexa that some days I eat bad food and today is that day without her thinking, "Oh sure, it's your 'day off'"? I'm being completely honest when I say that it was for sure my day off. At that time in my life, I was working promoting the show, so I usually chose a day I had off to have a cheat day. I told her this was my reset meal, and she was completely cool with it... another good sign.

One more thing that sticks out to me about that night was that Alexa managed to find a healthy meal in that stadium! I made an excuse not to eat healthy because we were surrounded by chili cheese fries and hot dogs. But Alexa was stronger than me. I love that she put her health first that night and continues to do so today. So many good signs from that night!

The game got rained out, so we all decided to go back to the bar we had met at only a few nights before.

I've been told I have a unique sense of humor. I would say it's just plain crude. But hey, that's me, and I own that. But I wasn't sure how Alexa would feel about it.

I thought about this as I went to the bathroom. I was still thinking about it when I walked up to the urinal to find that it was the tallest urinal I had ever seen. What the heck? These urinals were meant for Kareem Abdul-Jabbar. The guy is 7 feet 2 inches, and that's about how tall you would have to be to aim normally. For an average guy like myself, I had to shoot up, if you know what I mean.

When I returned, without thinking, I told Alexa all about my restroom experience. I had to be myself. And wouldn't you know it, she laughed her head off. She still says it's one of the funniest things she's ever heard on a first date. Apparently, I won her over as well.

The night was coming to a close. After so many good signs that night, I thought it was time to go in for a little kiss. I was nervous, but as soon as my lips met hers, I knew it was right. I'd never experienced a kiss like that before. I couldn't believe I went in for a kiss in public and it went so well.

After that night, I would never be alone again.

I never dreamed I'd find a woman as perfectly suited for me as she is. Alexa loves the color green, but not just any green. It's a mint green—a sea foam green. The shade suits her well because she has always reminded me of the sea. She is calm like the ocean waves. She is a constant source of light, like a lighthouse. She is hard-working, like a ship in the middle of a storm. She is a safe harbor. She is a bright horizon. And I want to sail into the sunset with her.

She is my wife now. Something that seemed unimaginable is a reality for me. In the past, I couldn't picture this kind of love being in my life. Have hope that good things are in your future just like they were for mine.

I spent so much time lamenting the fact that I would never find love. If I could've seen how perfectly it all worked out, I wouldn't have been anxious about anything. I work hard to have no regrets, but I've learned from my mistakes: Don't waste time worrying about what you don't have. Start working toward what you want, and you'll usually get it.

We don't get to see the future. We only get to live in the present. But one of my best pieces of advice is to be hopeful for good things to come into your life. There are amazing things in store for you! I know it! So keep pressing forward. Keep working on that goal. Keep imagining a good future, and one day you'll actually live it.

I LIKE TO SAY TO MYSELF

There's a good future. Just you wait.

Chapter 54

No Pain, No Pearls

D o you know how a pearl is formed? Well, don't worry, I didn't really understand the process either. It's truly fascinating, though. An oyster is going about, living its oyster life, when suddenly it gets injured. It's usually because of an attack from a parasite or a fish, which causes injury to the outer shell. It's through no fault of its own. In response to the trauma, the inside tissue begins secreting something called nacre into the pearl sack, and a cyst starts to form to heal the wound (I know, it all sounds very technical). Slowly, over time, the oyster heals, and a pearl is formed. It happens completely by chance.

But isn't that crazy? The oyster must first be hurt in order to create something beautiful. I have been hurt in my life. But once my body started the healing process, the end result was to receive not one pearl, but many pearls of wisdom. You can find your own pearls after any trial. All it takes is a little time. But you will find after every tribulation that there is a treasure to be found within yourself.

The pearl principle can apply to many areas of our lives. After the show, I wanted to keep making goals because it helps me a lot. Alexa is a big runner. I'm so proud of her for that. She signed up for a marathon... so I decided that I was going to run a marathon too. Everyone has their favorite flavor of working out and being active. For instance, my friend Bob Brenner is a real bike and yoga guy, but I love Cross-Fit and weights and all that. I knew running a marathon was going to be a challenge for me, but I was up for it. Heck yeah, baby! But because I don't naturally gravitate toward running every day, my training was... not as good as it could've been. But you know by now that I'm a big fan of having integrity, and that means keeping promises. So with very little training, I ran the marathon. I'm not going to lie, it wasn't easy. But I finished!

I cannot describe how my legs felt the next day. I had depleted every reserve within my body, and I had broken down every muscle. I hurt, man. I hurt bad. My legs felt like jelly. I was like the oyster that had been broken down. But because I did that marathon, I grew stronger physically in the weeks that followed. I could run farther and do more. I will never run a full marathon again, but I've participated in half marathons and continued to work on my cardio game.

This process of breaking down in order to form something beautiful is the same for weightlifting. You have to slightly tear the tissues of your muscles in order for them to grow back bigger than before. I'm not suggesting you hurt yourself. There is a smart way to lift weights and make gains. Always be careful and smart about it. But truly, when you're packing on the muscle, you have to almost traumatize the existing muscle.

My whole life feels like an oyster. It's been messy. The rough waves have crashed over me. Extreme trauma has affected me. But I got a pearl out of it. I'm not afraid to say it. And it's awesome and beautiful. It feels great and I'm so blessed.

I LIKE TO SAY TO MYSELF

Setbacks create pearls.

Chapter 55

It's All About YOU

True humility is not thinking less of yourself;
it is thinking of yourself less.

—*C. S. Lewis*

I t's hard to admit, but for a long time I was only thinking about myself. I tried my best to be a good son, a good friend, and a good person. I wanted to be kind to others. But I think sometimes I was doing it for the wrong reasons. I developed strong insecurities because of my dad's lack of dad-ness, basically. So while deep down I cared about other people, I also just really wanted them to like me. I wanted their acceptance. It makes me feel stupid to say it now because what I didn't know was that I already had their love. And if I asked the people who are close to you in your life how they felt about you, you would hear that they only have love for you too.

The path toward losing the weight and living life free from the burdens that hold you back is packed full of truths that will smack you in the face. There are things that you have to look at that will hurt. It's good to be positive. I believe in positive rewards and getting better through being inspired. But, un-fortunately, there are some things about the process that are going to make you uncomfortable. I don't say this to scare you or discourage you, but to prepare you. Pain doesn't have to be something to fear. Embrace the pain! Without pain, there is no gain. And eventually, when you realize you have nothing to worry about, those unpleasant feelings will subside.

One truth that hurt me the most was that by being over-weight, I was not keeping my integrity. I was not being the best version of myself. I was being selfish. To *not* lose weight was hurting others. Loving others is about being the best you can be. When I was 400 pounds, there was no way I was doing that. When you're overweight, you're being weighed down by burdens and most of the time it becomes hard to focus on anything else. You become a slave to your own thoughts. You might be able to fake it around people, but deep down it's all you think about. Even though you don't want to, or may not be able to recognize it, you're only thinking about yourself.

I did that. I did that big time. Before the show, when I hung out with my friends, I would always apologize. If I spilled something. If I was late. If I said something I thought might upset them. I was constantly saying I was sorry. It's good to accept blame when you've done something wrong. But I was doing it so often that it was really just a cry for ac-ceptance and a sign of poor self-esteem. I apologized all the time because I didn't think I was good enough. My friends would always say something like, "Oh, it's okay, Bruce. Don't worry about it." In a small way, their forgiveness made me feel better. This whole cycle of apologizing and receiving for-giveness was my life. The more my friends would build me up, the more I worried about having to be built up all the time. I thought I was a burden. Then I would apologize for being a burden. On and on and on. I was so focused on myself because I didn't know how not to be.

But there is a way to free yourself and your mind from this: Focus on others. When you start thinking about other people, you begin to forget your own problems, and soon you realize your problems are solvable anyway. When you focus on other people, you can see where they are struggling, and you can help them. Everyone is going through something. Take the time to get to know them and learn what they might need help with. Part of the reason I did so well on the show was because I liked cheering for the other contestants. I liked helping them. If I saw them lagging, I would run back and help them. If I knew they were hurting, I would push through my own pain to show them it was possible.

On your saddest day, try reaching out to a friend who you know is going through a hard time. Send them a text or call them to see how they're doing. Buy them a small gift or invite them for a workout. It might not make your sadness go away entirely, but I guarantee it will help shift your focus. Knowing that other people are also struggling puts your own struggles in perspective. We are all in this world together. When you give of yourself, it will come back tenfold, I promise you.

Because that's the beauty of it all. Helping others helps you too. While it stings, I know my friends thought of me as a burden at times. And that's because I was a burden! I used to always call them, going on about this or that. But now they are the ones calling me. I am a new man. They want workout tips or advice. I leaned on them for so many years, and now they're leaning on me sometimes.

Go out there and think about someone else. You'll get your weight off. You'll restore what was lost. You'll live a good life.

Don't worry about any of that. Think about the friend you know who needs someone. We all have to take turns being there for one another.

I LIKE TO SAY TO MYSELF

Take turns leaning on each other.

Chapter 56

Barbells and Wedding Bells

The morning of our wedding, I felt so at peace. I had just had a great bachelor party with all of my friends. We partied hard, and it was awesome. We decided to have our wedding in Colorado because that's where Alexa is from. Alexa and I had already relocated to Utah, so we flew in for the big day.

Having all my closest friends in one place was enough to make my heart burst. I didn't feel nervous, just excited to finally marry the girl of my dreams. I wanted to spend the whole morning just basking in that feeling. But I knew I had to rise and grind because when you've transformed into a new you, you don't take a day off.

By the end of your weight-loss journey, you will be a new person. You will have so many tools, and your thought process about life will be different. Your mind, body, and soul will all be transformed. But it's strange because that old you is still a memory. If you think about how you used to be, it can be easy to fall back into past behaviors. In the past, I didn't work out every day. I didn't eat clean every day. I didn't work on my emotional health and check my feelings every day. I certainly wouldn't have done any of that on my wedding day. But the morning I got married, instead of being the old me, I chose to continue to be the new me. That is why I made sure to get a workout in before saying "I do."

Because that's who I am. I'm a guy who works out on his wedding day. I love it. The craziest part of all is that I *wanted* to work out. So my fourteen groomsmen, Chris, and I worked out with some of my other buddies. (It's hard to believe I still had friends who weren't groomsmen!) We had a blast.

You can't be someone part of the time. You have to be authentic and live that way 24/7. Once you have lost the weight, never think you're done. Instead, think of your whole life as a journey. Truly understanding that I can never go back to where I was is a big part of my continual growth. It's front and center.

I got my workout in that morning and proceeded to experience the best day of my life. It was a perfect day.

I LIKE TO SAY TO MYSELF

This is a new life. Live it 24/7.

Chapter 57

Faith

*Without the assistance of that Divine Being, I
cannot succeed. With that assistance, I cannot fail.*
—*Abraham Lincoln*

I believe in God. It's religion that is a bit trickier for me. I have never doubted that there is a higher power. And while it has definitely wavered at times, I have always had faith. I was raised as a Mormon, and I still consider myself to be Mormon. But my definition of what that means has shifted.

I've already talked a lot about growing up Mormon. We went to church every Sunday, but beyond that, we didn't do much. However, it should be no surprise that my father was a "deeply" religious man. Unlike me, my dad completed his mission—my mom did too. He would talk about what a great Mormon he was. He had "proof" too, rising in the ranks of leadership at our church. Everyone there thought he was a strong example of what a good Mormon should be. He prayed for people and fulfilled all of his church duties like it was nothing. He appeared to be a good, religious guy. One time at home, we got these cartoon videos that help

213

guide you through reading the *Book of Mormon*. My dad and I would watch it together, just the two of us. It's taken me a long time to reconcile my father's God with my own. Now I can see that there is a big difference.

They say that your image of God is similar to your earthly father. I know in some ways that was true for me. I used to think God was disappointed in me and that I didn't deserve His love. Just like how I felt around my actual dad, I felt like I was worthless in God's eyes. Nothing could convince me that I was worthy. I had failed my mission, after all. Your mission is supposed to be two years of your life that you give to Christ for all He's done for you. What did that mean for me? I thought I deserved to be punished.

But now I see things a whole lot differently. God is the one you can turn to when everything else falls away. He's never angry with me or disappointed in me. He has blessings for me to be successful. I don't believe in coincidences. Everything happens for a reason. These all sound like taglines, but they are for sure true. God gives me tools to get through trials and adversities. My mom says that all the blessings for our family are coming now. And I believe that.

If you believe and have faith, God will give to you too. We all have our own trials. Each trial is just as hard for the individual who's going through it. But having faith will get you through it. It helps. Trust me.

While you may not be a part of an organized religion, having faith is critical to your success. Knowing there is something greater than yourself—looking out for you—is a powerful thing. No matter how good they can be or how loving their intentions are, people will fail you. They will let you down. I don't say this to discourage you, I just love to talk in truths. But there is a God who will never fail you. He is always there for you, even when no one else is. Having faith in something that is pure love, well, that's a beautiful thing. Faith has the power to transform your life because it allows you to hope for the future. Faith is believing something that hasn't happened yet. Faith is seeing yourself fit, happy, and healthy even though you're still wearing size 5X pants.

The first part of weight loss and a new life is believing you will succeed. You've got to have a voice in your head that says you will reach that goal. It's a mindset. And the reason I stress faith so much is because if you believe you will lose the weight, but don't believe in a God or a higher power, then what are you believing in?

I LIKE TO SAY TO MYSELF

Have faith.

Chapter 58

Forgiveness

My life has changed in so many ways since my show aired in June 2014. Good and bad, it's all been for the better. It was the gift of a lifetime. But one of the strangest things since I lost the weight is that people seem to ask me the same question over and over again, "Bruce, what's your secret?" I don't mind. I'm just not used to people asking me, a former fat kid from Provo, for advice. When I go to speaking engagements, or when I'm working out at the gym, I'm approached by people who are in the same place I was a few years ago. They look at me as if I have some golden ticket, or that I know where the tree of life is located. All of them want to know how I did it. What was that special thing I did that made everything work? What was my secret to success?

I'm going to tell you the biggest secret of all: There is no secret. There is no magic bean or catchphrase that will be a quick fix. Changing your life is a million little adjustments to every aspect of your mind, body, and spirit. There is not one, singular tool that will fix everything. It doesn't happen overnight. Transforming into a new you takes a massive amount of hard work.

Plus, I don't keep secrets anymore. That's why I wanted to write this book. I wanted to share all of the knowledge I have. My success has been built from the foundational ideas in each chapter. The things I use every day—the things I repeat to myself to help me stay on this path—are all in this book.

All that being said, I did save the best tool I possess for last. It is the cornerstone for the entire process. And it's also the most difficult tool to acquire and use. Out of all I've learned about exercise, diet, and mental and emotional health, without this one thing, I wouldn't have been able to get where I am and be who I am today.

You cannot take one more step forward in your journey without this. It is the foundation you will build off of for your entire life. It's the cement slab on which you build the entire house.

I'm talking about forgiveness. Forgiving is the hardest thing you'll ever do. But it will free you to live your life with peace. Forgiveness is vital to the success of your life.

Buddha said, "Holding on to anger is like drinking poison and expecting the other person to die." There is so much truth in that.

Forgiveness brings about such an amazing new life that it's insane that more people hang on to bitterness, resentment, and anger instead. For years I was like that. It's because it's easier to live in a negative place. The pessimist always wins. There's also a certain entitlement to your negative feelings. You think you're allowed to be upset forever because someone really did wrong you. There will be many moments in life when you are completely screwed over and you didn't deserve it. There are mean people out there who will tear you down for no reason at all, other than the fact that they have some darkness in their own life. Look, it's easier to forgive someone who recognizes their behavior, apologizes, and asks for forgiveness. But if you're waiting for that, you'll usually be waiting forever. When we hope for the wrongdoer to change, it does no good. In the highly unlikely event that they do, our problems may go away, but we will have learned nothing. Without learning and forgiving, there is no change; and without change, there is no growth. Instead, we must forgive so our own spirit can become like water: Water has the ability to flow through and over the toughest obstacles but also to be completely still. Water is cleansing. Water brings growth. Forgive and flow like water.

Forgiveness takes an incredible amount of strength, yet it happens in an instant. Letting go will have the most profound effect on your entire life.

The year I was on the show was also the year of my dad's parole hearing. He had served fifteen years of his sentence. Now it was up to the board to decide whether he would stay in prison longer or be released. I knew from the very first day of filming that his hearing would be coming up, but as the days leading up to it grew nearer, I didn't know if I could confront him. I would work out and think about it constantly. What would I say? Could I say anything at all? I wanted to speak at the hearing. I wanted to put all of that behind me, but the day was rapidly approaching, and I didn't know what to do.

The day of my dad's parole hearing, I was a mess. I can't describe it. No amount of preparation could've fully equipped me for that moment. The friends and family who came and sat beside me will forever be my heroes. Everyone had different feelings that day. So many emotions were swirling around. I still didn't know if I would say anything in front of the board. Some of the producers who had become close friends told me that I needed to say something. But seeing how shaken up I was, Heidi came in like a mama hen and comforted me. She said, "You don't have to say anything if you don't want to."

When we entered the courtroom, my heart stopped. My dad was sitting, facing the judge, with his back to us. That's how they do it with sex offenders. They don't let them look their victims in eye. I could barely look at the back of him. Heidi was feeling intensely empathetic, but Chris was feeling angry. He has said since, "Honestly, God could snatch the life out of him and I would probably sleep better." Chris had trouble with my dad. What my dad did to innocent children sparks a really deep anger in him. I don't blame him. Chris is a father of four. When the judge read the charges, Chris got more and more angry. But I was overwhelmed. I started physically shaking and crying. There was no hiding, no escaping my past. Here it was being read aloud. My dad's family was sitting across the aisle glaring at me. But immediately surrounding me was my own family, both blood relatives and friends that had become my family. The people that loved me with real love.

After the accusations were read, the hearing went on. All my dad had to say was, "I'm very proud of both my sons. They mean a lot to me." How was that even possible? When asked if he abused me, after a long and lengthy answer, my dad said, "No." At that point Chris had enough. He said he felt sick. I had many feelings that are too hard to describe. But I knew what I had to do. I had to speak. I didn't write anything down. I didn't know what I would say. But when the judge asked me if I would like to share, I knew I had to do it. That's what I had worked for. That's what I was there for. The words just came to me, but I had trouble getting them

out. Facing the person who stole most of my life from me
made me weak in a way that I had never been weak before.
Through many tears, I managed to say:

> I did love my dad with all my heart. I thought he was
> the greatest thing ever. I did so many things to try and
> make him happy. I wanted to be that son. It kills me
> to say this—and I'm sorry, Dad—but I don't think he
> should get out. It's hard for me to say it; I just believe
> that's what needs to happen for his safety and every-
> body else's. I just want to make a stand for all the vic-
> tims and let them know that it's okay to confront the
> person who did it to you.

And just like that, I was free. It was all over.

Chris said that when I spoke, everything changed for him:
"Bruce spoke with such love and forgiveness and kindness
and compassion. He came from such a place of love that it
made me walk out of there a different person." Heidi said,
"[Bruce] is like this ray of sunshine and love. The cold, dark
courtroom became warm, and lit, and happy, and understanding." Skyler said the moment was overwhelming. To
have all the people that I love and admire the most say those
things about me is truly humbling. I wouldn't have been able
to do it without them.

Chris took it one step further and said something about
me that I don't think is true, though. He said I was about as
Christ-like as it gets. I'm no savior but there are times when
I feel like I was as innocent as a little lamb. Then I was sacri-
ficed and came out clean on the other side.

There's a person in your life that you need to forgive.
Maybe you have a grudge against someone. Take the time

you need, and only act when you are ready, but eventually you will be able to do it. You will be able to forgive and move forward. If you're struggling to think of a person you need to forgive, maybe it's because the person you need to forgive is yourself. I had to forgive my dad, but I also had to forgive myself. I had to let go of the judgment I put on myself for getting so big. It's the hardest thing, but when you forgive yourself, then you can accept that everything is okay.

I LIKE TO SAY TO MYSELF

Forgiveness is freedom.

Chapter 59

A New Beginning

My dad got life in prison. After the parole hearing, my dad didn't have control over me anymore. People are always talking about one thing changing their whole life. That's exactly what happened to me. Once I got up and spoke to my dad, the weight of my entire life was lifted from my shoulders. Before that, my dad was always on my mind. His voice was always in my head. I was never good enough. But after the parole hearing, my dad's voice vanished. I don't need his approval. I am who I am. I have a new life. I feel like everything is just beginning.

I find great strength in the bible verse Genesis 50:20, "You intended to harm me, but God intended it for good to accomplish what is now being done, the saving of many lives."

The events in my past will always be a part of my life, but now I can honestly say that they don't control me. I'm not weighed down by them. All that remains are the good things I've gained because of them. I know it sounds crazy that a nightmare can turn into a weird fairy tale. But that's my life.

Overcoming my dad's abuse feels like I won the Super Bowl. And my new body feels like the Lombardi Trophy.

Losing my weight has given me a new body, but losing my emotional weight has given me a new life. Take it from me—you can have a new life too. I don't even know you, but I believe in you. You got this. Get pumped, baby!

I WILL ALWAYS SAY TO MYSELF

Get pumped!

ACKNOWLEDGMENTS

First, I would like to thank my backbone, my heart, my life, my wife: Alexa Pitcher. You have given me unconditional love and have been my strongest supporter every step of the way. I want to thank my mom, Janet Pitcher, and my brother, Brandon. You two are my blood. Thank you to Alexa's family, who are now my family. Chris and Heidi Powell, you are my family too. Thank you for guiding me through not only my weight loss, but my life every day after. Thank you to my uncle Johnny and my aunt Joyce Pitcher and your family. You guys were in my corner when it really mattered.

Thank you to all my friends that I met growing up. Thank you, Bailey Wood, for helping me through one of the hardest times of my life. Thank you, Corey Seiuli and Chad Vanoder. Thank you, Skyler Strong and the entire Strong family for being just like your last name. To Nick Jones and his family, thank you.

A huge thank you to all my coaches: Coach Olson and family, Coach Wong, Coach Clark and family, Coach Walker, and all the coaches I've ever had. You've all left a positive, lasting impression on my life. You fed me spiritually, mentally, and literally! Coaches lead a team, and I want to thank all my teammates as well. Thank you to every single player who stepped on the field with me.

High school was such a crazy time in my life, so I want to thank all the teachers, close friends, and church members who were there for me.

Thank you, Todd Pederson, for betting on me.

Thank you to ABC for giving me the opportunity and ultimately saving my life. Thank you, J. D. Roth, Jason Kemp, Hagar Elaziz, Lisa Stanley, Serina Stelamire (my rock), Matt Assmus, and all the producers on the show. Thank you to all the crew behind the scenes. Thank you, Rob Whittaker, for making me look so dang good on camera. And no doubt, I have to thank John Ball. Thank you to all the trainers, counselors, and doctors on the show, especially Dr. Holly. And to all of the experts who fixed my smile and my skin, thank you! Donielle, you took care of all of us. I don't know what we would've done without you. Thank you.

ABC's *Extreme Weight Loss* introduced me to the other competitors who would be huge supports to me on and off the show. Thank you, Bob Brenner. I'm forever grateful the show connected us. To my horsemen Jayce, David, and Rod, I give thanks for you all every day. Rod, I miss you, man. Thank you to all the contestants on my season, and all the seasons before and after.

To all the guys I've met since the show—Jake Hutton, Tommy Hackenbruck, Mike Cazayoux—you guys inspire me every day. I never dreamed I would get to meet guys like you. Thank you for helping me crush it. Thank you, Project Rise. It's always nice to have a place to work out that feels like home. Thank you, Alex Takacs.

Thank you, Caleb Sommer, for believing in me enough to manage this project. And to Meredith Smith, thank you for editing and bringing it all together. Thank you, Jan and Matt

Sommer. Thank you, Rachel Sommer, for capturing my life in words.

I have to thank my Raiders! Having your team to root for has been a source of constant comfort in my life. Even on my darkest days, I know I have my Raiders.

It is frustrating that I can't list every single person that I want to thank. So I'll throw out one more thank you to everyone: Thank you.

Lastly, I want to thank God. Through Him all things are possible.

RESOURCES

MENTAL HEALTH AND ABUSE

Better Help
betterhelp.com

National Suicide Prevention Lifeline
1-800-273-TALK
suicidepreventionlifeline.org

National Sexual Assault Hotline
(run by RAINN, Rape, Abuse & Incest National Network)
1-800-656-HOPE
hotline.rainn.org

Lifeline Crisis Chat
contact-usa.org/chat.html

1in6
1in6.org

EXERCISE AND NUTRITION

Transform with Chris and Heidi
thetransformapp.com

12 Week Transformation Challenge
brucepitcher.pages.ontraport.net

Project Rise
projectrisefitness.com

The Plant Paradox
Dr. Steven Gundry

Extreme Transformation
Chris and Heidi Powell

Working Against Gravity
workingagainstgravity.com

University of Colorado Anschutz Health and Wellness
Center
anschutzwellness.com

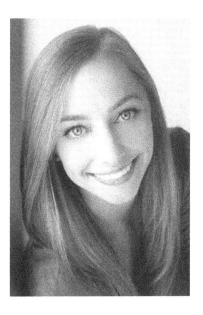

Rachel Sommer is an independent screenwriter and a creative developer for the production company Whisperstone Productions, run by her family. She lives with her tricolored collie, Wynnie, in southern California.

CPSIA information can be obtained
at www.ICGtesting.com
Printed in the USA
FFHW021918291218
50005787-54739FF